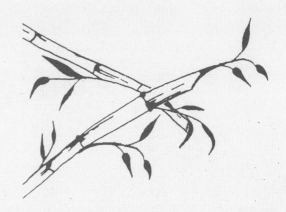

Pamela Hannay 1949–2001

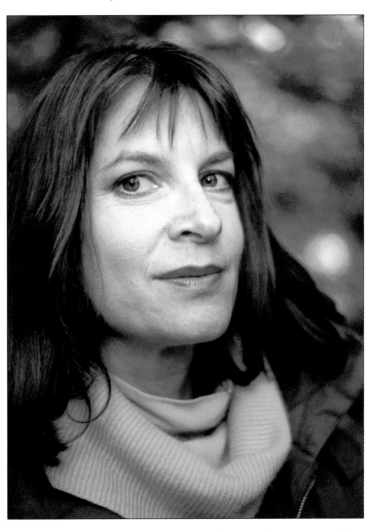

who teaches us to live

SHIATSU THERAPY FOR HORSES

Know your horse and yourself better through shiatsu

PAMELA HANNAY

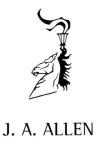

J. A. ALLEN

ISBN 0 85131 847 9

J. A. Allen
Clerkenwell House
Clerkenwell Green
London EC1R 0HT

J. A. Allen is an imprint of Robert Hale Ltd

British Library Cataloguing in Publication Data
A catalogue record for this book is available from the British Library

Disclaimer
The techniques in this book are not intended to replace veterinary diagnosis
and treatment. The author and publisher cannot be held responsible for any
injury resulting from the performance of these techniques. It is assumed that the
reader be well versed in safe horse handling and will take full responsibility for
the risks in working around large animals whose first instinct is flight.

Design by Nancy Lawrence
Illustrated by Peggy Fleming DVM
Photographs by Adrian Buckmaster
Edited by Jane Lake
Colour separation by Tenon & Polert Colour Scanning Ltd
Printed by Kyodo Printing Co., Singapore

Contents

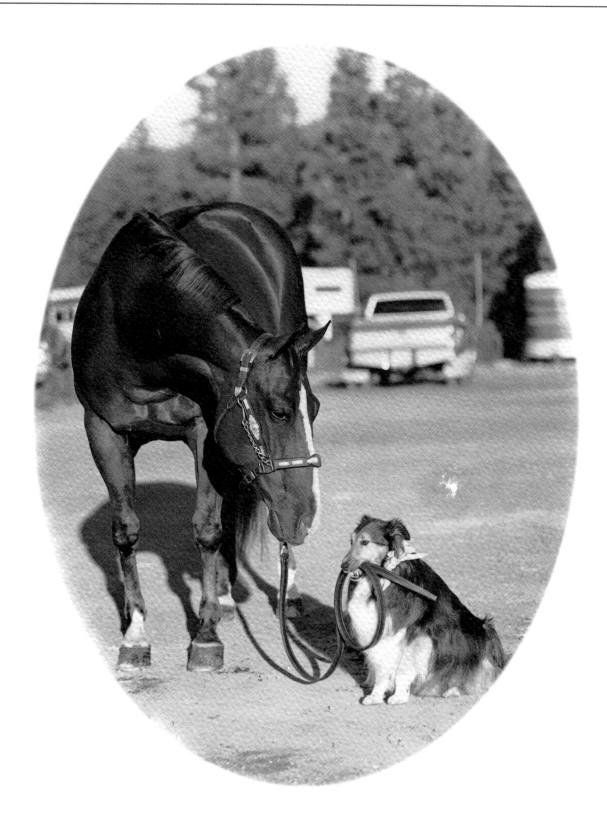

Waiting for Pamela
(photograph by Lyle Orson)

FOR MY DAUGHTER
WHO LOVES ANIMALS

by Dorianne Laux

Once a week, whether the money is there
or not, I write a check for her lessons.
But today, as I waited in the car for her
to finish her chores, after she had wrapped
this one's delicate legs, brushed burrs
and caked mud from that one's tail,
I saw her stop and offer her body
to a horse's itchy head. One arm up,
she gave him the whole length of her side.
And he knew the gesture, understood
the gift, stepped in close on oiled hooves
and pressed his head to her ribcage.
From hip to armpit he raked her body until,
to keep from falling, she leaned into him
full weight, her foot braced
against a tack post for balance.
Before horses, it was snakes, coiled
around her arms like African bracelets.
And before that, stray dogs, cats
of every color, even the misfits,
the abandoned and abused.
It took me so long to learn how to love,
how to give myself up and over to another.
Now I see how she has always
loved them all, snails and spiders,
from the very beginning, without fear or shame,
saw even the least of them, ants,
gnats, heard and answered
even the slightest of their calls.

Acknowledgements

I wish to thank Adrian Buckmaster, my fabulous photographer and dear friend. Adrian embraced this project with enthusiasm for horses and support of my work. Special appreciation to Phyllis Baker who assisted me during the photography days by grooming, handling, holding tails out of the way and making sure she stayed invisible; her presence was supportive and calming to all.

My thanks to Lyle Orson for the frontispiece photograph 'Waiting for Pamela'.

Thank you to Peggy Fleming DVM for her generosity in allowing her excellent illustrations to appear in this book.

I thank Nancy Wolff for my main model, Cameron, (Percheron, Thoroughbred cross, 16.3 hh), a retired eventer. He evented at novice and training level, was driven, and is now teaching younger horses and giving lessons. Nancy was generous in allowing me to do most of the photos at her beautiful facility in Califon, New Jersey.

Thanks to Jane Suwalsky, owner of Neruda (Nobel, 17.3 hh); his sire, Haarlem, is a Dutch Warmblood and his dam's sire is Ladalco. Rudy is just beginning to do dressage competitions; he is the tall horse model and appears on the cover.

Thank you to my friend Debbie Lloyd who owns Rocky, the model for the face techniques; Rocky is a mixed breed horse. Thank you also to Emily and Sylvester, Jacqui and Cinnamon, Debbie's daughters and their horses.

Thank you to Jacqueline Cook, owner of Russell, the Shetland. He was bought from Sheffield Animal Sanctuary as a two-year-old, for five pounds. Russell is an extremely accomplished pony who has received regular shiatsu for years. He is a Midlands Driving Trials Group Intermediate pony. In the 1999 season he was driven at Intermediate Level where he won three out of five dressage tests and placed second and third in the remaining tests which a Shetland has never done at the Intermediate level before. He went on to be placed in the top three of the other two phases of driving trials. He has won many rosettes, trophies and shields in pleasure driving classes.

Jacqueline Cook, who is the sister of my heart, has promoted my work extensively. True teachers want their students to learn and then surpass them. This woman will do so. I wish to thank Jacqueline's husband, Peter

Cook, who is a good friend and the energy behind the scenes that has helped make my courses in Great Britain successful. With great humor and kindness, Peter is an invaluable support and is also a good photographer; he took the photos of me working on the pony.

I thank Maureen Miller, my special friend and colleague, who modeled for the partner stretches. She is a senior instructor at the Ohashi Institute. Maureen walks in beauty.

Caroline Burt, my publisher and friend, is a smart and lovely lady. She has been patient and supportive through thick and thin. Caroline has always been there for me. Her vision and love of horses has given me the exposure I have dreamed of. Jane Lake, my editor, has a way with words. She has been an enthusiastic supporter of shiatsu for dogs and horses, is a beautiful person and a unique individual. Thank you to Nancy Lawrence for her creative book design.

Thank you to Nancie and Ed Giblock who gave my husband and me a great honor in asking us to be godparents to their daughter Alisa. She is our darling girl.

To my friends who share their children with me, thank you. Timmy, Nick and Jessica are children of my heart. I am truly blessed by these big hearts in little bodies. There are many other little ones who enrich my life with love and laughter.

My love and appreciation go to my family at the Ohashi Institute.

Dr. Anusak Yiengpruksawan, my brillant surgeon, has hands and a heart of gold. He really cares.

Bless you Dr. Haim Bicher, director of Valley Cancer Institute in Los Angeles, California, for giving me the chance to give more love to the world. All doctors should have such compassion.

Thank you Sylvia Carter, also of Valley Cancer Institute, for your open heart, beautiful spirit, keen wit and bountiful love.

Thank you Tony Carlson of Digital Boss for the expertise and professionalism in creating meridian lines by computer.

Linda Munato, who keeps my house clean and her prayers flowing, has been a huge help to me for many years. Linda's confidence in me is appreciated.

My parents, Francine and Howard Hannay, have shown me harmony between two people. They have been beyond supportive, especially during my recent difficult time. My sister Michelle, a beautiful and multi-talented woman, keeps me laughing.

Dot Larsen and Gladys Hollowell, precious friends and aunties of my heart.

Dick and Marge Aschoff, my husband's parents, are the in-laws that women only dream of. I love them dearly. My brother-in-law, Steven, is my bro, and a big, gorgeous blessing.

To all my students, who keep me growing.

My husband, Richard Aschoff, is my best friend, soul mate and conscience. He tries to keep my feet on the ground. He is the yang to my yin.

I am so blessed in my life that I am able to let so much love surround me.

Dedication

To those who have learned to listen to the profound silence.

Part I

PREPARATION

Introduction

This book will guide you into a world of improved understanding and communication with your horse, and perhaps other animals and humans. Touching techniques have been used for thousands of years to comfort and heal with great success. In our present modern day world of the quick fix, touch comes often as a last resort, when medicines and surgery have weakened the patient. There are more and more people who understand that touching therapies are valid and necessary and, when employed in an educated and heartfelt manner, may accomplish miraculous results. These techniques and theories are not intended to replace modern technology but to enhance these therapies and give the horse owner/handler a greater capacity to help the animals in their care.

Shiatsu is a healing art, and therefore subject to individual interpretation. There are many styles that have been developed by many masters of the art. The style in which I work has been influenced by my first teachers. Wataru Ohashi has brilliantly developed a unique form of shiatsu, called Ohashiatsu. This style focuses on the balanced use of the practitioner's body, and the harmony achieved between two partners during a session. I have been teaching Ohashiatsu for twenty-three years, since 1979, and admire the style and philosophy tremendously. It has helped me to stay healthy and happy, and has been a springboard to my work with animals. Also a valuable influence on my work was Master Shizuto Masunaga, who came to America each year when I first began my studies. He developed an extended meridian system, the personality of the meridians, and helped us to look at ourselves and understand how we develop tendencies toward certain health issues.

Traditional Western medicine developed to treat disease and its symptoms, without necessarily looking at the individual. Today, this view is changing, with many physicians learning and practicing certain forms of Asian medicine. This change is happening too slowly. With increasing use of drug therapy, body systems are becoming weaker as the side effects of drugs are often more troubling than the original complaint. Drugs are becoming more sophisticated and are better able to target the disease without harming the rest of the body but one important fact remains: we are not getting healthier. We and the animals in our care must often struggle to recreate good health and equilibrium after the disease has been cured. It is the individual's responsibility to understand the limitations of modern medicine and take steps to support health and prevent disease.

Most disease begins with subtle symptoms. These symptoms do not necessarily fit into the mold of a particular disease. The homeopathic or naturopathic practitioner may be able to help the patient at this point. The acupuncturist or shiatsu practitioner may also help the body recover balance before the symptoms become more advanced. These and other natural practitioners ask many questions of the client, to understand the tendency of the individual to develop these symptoms, and help direct the client toward some lifestyle changes. It is frustrating and unsatisfactory when a doctor or veterinarian is unable to diagnose illness until it becomes a blatant problem. Then, of course, the patient has become weak, both physically and mentally, and the natural tendency to heal has begun to be compromised. Many times, even though the disease has been cured, the patient dies because of the inability to recover from the devastating effect of the drugs that have been responsible for the cure. While the drugs attack the invading organism or disease, they also attack the healthy parts.

We must learn how to take intelligent responsibility for our bodies and those of the animals in our care. The ability for self-healing is tremendous. The body 'wants' to be whole. There are so many avenues available to those who look. The alternative therapies may take longer than conventional medicine but, in the long haul, they support our health rather than compromise it. When treated early with gentle remedies, the body can become even healthier than before the first symptoms made themselves known. It is easier to take a drug to repress symptoms, and sometimes may even be appropriate to temporarily relieve the emotionally stressful signals of illness, but the dependence on these remedies weakens our immune systems. Fever is the mechanism for burning out an invading organism and should not automatically be brought down, but when your child is burning up in the middle of the night, it is a difficult and often dangerous decision to let it 'run its course'.

Children of the Western world are mostly stuffed with medicine to buffer the symptoms brought on by chemicals in their environment. These dangerous chemicals are in the air, food additives, cleaning agents and disposable diapers. Respiratory ailments in children are epidemic. It is unusual for a child not to have been on a course of antibiotics during the first year of life.

How many horses have never been on phenylbutazone because the owner knows that even though the symptoms may be temporarily masked, the complaint is still there? An ache or pain is the body's signal that something is wrong. If we ignore these signals, eventually something that modern medicine can name will develop. Holistic treatments are effective for treating the individual before diseases have been named, as well as afterward. They seek to restore the individual to a state of glowing health, rather than bring about only the abatement of disease. In the hectic lifestyle most people lead, symptoms may not even be noticed until they are quite pronounced. We must become more sensitive to ourselves and to others, as well as to our environment.

I have been developing techniques for horses since 1983. Many of the techniques in the book *Touching Horses* are augmented for better results and easier applications. My focus in *Shiatsu Therapy for Horses* is to not only help your horses, but also to create more strength and balance in your own body. I will stress the use of your body in a balanced and mindful way so you may feel stronger and more energized after each session than before, so that whatever activities you engage in may be performed with more ease and flow and balance and, of course, more enjoyment. It is my desire that you should be happy and healthy along with your horses, and that these techniques in some way contribute to that end.

There are four chapters devoted solely to the bodies of people. The meridian stretches, done alone or with a partner, will help you understand your body in terms of energy, as well as muscles, tendons and ligaments. They may help somewhat in self-diagnosis. For example, you might notice that the Lung and Large Intestine Meridian stretch is more difficult on a particular day. It may happen that you have a cold developing. Before the actual symptoms begin, you could start taking some natural remedies and get some rest. Or, if you have difficulty doing the Stomach and Spleen Meridian stretch, you may not have been taking very good care of your eating habits, and the tightness in the stretch is a good reminder to be gentler with yourself. The partner stretching is fun, and a good way to help each other. The feedback from your partner will help confirm to you that you are becoming more flexible. The self-shiatsu is relaxing, healing and diagnostic as well.

The preride exercises will simultaneously center, stretch, and strengthen your body, promoting balance. I developed them with the particular demands of riding in mind. The exercises will promote awareness, and should benefit the body of the rider; no matter what discipline he or she practices.

I have been developing this style of Shiatsu to 'fit' the combination of human with horse, no matter what their relative sizes are. My students who are practicing these techniques regularly tell me that their awareness in many other areas of life becomes attuned. They slow down and take in the finer details. Their individual relationships become enhanced. I am moved and touched by descriptions of how my teachings have brought happiness and health to people and animals.

Giving a shiatsu session fosters healing in both partners. The treatment itself is a moving meditation. The concentration of the practitioner can be profound. Horse and human become intertwined in a dance. This is a dance of celebration of the energy that is life. When the giver connects with the energy of the horse, the session flows and there is no intellectual decision guiding the work; it is pure instinct and joy.

The practitioner becomes a channel for healing. I do not believe that the practitioner is using his or her own energy to give to the horse during a session, but becomes a channel or catalyst for healing. An individual would need to have a tremendous amount of purely healthy energy to be able to share it, and this energy would need to be in a perpetual state of clarity and abundance. I prefer to believe that the therapist is so clear and open a channel, so healthy and centered, that energy flows through his or her body as needed with nothing getting 'stuck' going in either direction. Even if the technical aspect is not perfect, the person with compassion in his or her hands can accomplish marvelous results.

As a channel for healing energy, we do not need to consider the possibility of picking up 'bad energy' from another individual. When asked if he thought we could pick up bad energy from someone, Master Shizuto Masunaga replied, 'If you think you can, you will'. Thus, it becomes enormously important for the practitioner to have a system of self-healing, to be able to stay open and healthy and to be a good catalyst for helping others. This is why I encourage my students to eat well, exercise and meditate regularly, and learn how to deal gracefully with stressful situations. A total immersion into a healthy lifestyle (without becoming a boring fanatic) is vital for the successful practitioner.

The healing that occurs during a session comes from outside the giver, and goes through the giver. This healing energy can be viewed by the practitioner according to her or his own personal belief system. It could be thought of as God's love, universal energy, prana, ki, or chi, energy, as well as other aspects of energetic healing. Calling yourself a 'healer' may be viewed negatively by certain portions of the population. We are all healers and all have the potential to foster healing in others and ourselves. It is important for each individual to find the modality that resonates within, that feels natural and healthy, that works for each unique person.

Another observation I greatly appreciate from Master Masunaga is why the vertical pressure of shiatsu feels good. He explained that during gestation, we are surrounded by amniotic fluid, which is vertical pressure all over our bodies. After birth this comfortable and comforting pressure is suddenly gone and we miss it. Therefore, one reason shiatsu feels so 'right' is that it exerts direct vertical pressure on the body.

There are many healing modalities to study and, with attention to detail and a good heart, all will work to some degree. We need the choice of a varied approach since so many problems are many faceted. The horse owner needs to be aware of the many healing modalities so that he or she can make an educated decision, or at least not have to try everything while the problem continues to worsen. Fortunately, the alternatives for the most part do no harm and most will help, at least to some degree. When asked why there were so many healing modalities, Master Masunaga replied, 'Because there is such a variety of problems'.

Shiatsu is so versatile and works on a variety of levels. It is a perfect body, mind, spirit, approach. The educated practitioner can uncover aspects of the horse that the long-time owner may not be aware of. In the process of observing the horse and working on him, the shiatsu therapist may be able to inform the horse owner not only where the pains are, but also explain why the personality quirks that have occurred since the physical problems began are understandable. The practitioner will also be able, through touch, to eliminate the behaviour problems that are associated with physical discomfort. Even the beginner will gain an understanding of the horse not before imagined. Long-term relationships will be enhanced and deepened.

The thing that inspires me and fills me with awe is that doing shiatsu means I am literally touching life. This is an honor and joy that I pay respect to before, during and after each treatment on human, horse or dog. I feel particularly alive when I do shiatsu.

Dr. George Goodheart, the father of applied kineseology, said 'when you're on fire with an idea, people will come from miles away to watch you burn'. After so many years of interacting with this work, I am still burning with enthusiasm.

Touch

Since the publication of the book *Touching Horses*, many wonderful people have come to study with me. I am honored to be with these people who have the strong desire to deepen their relationship with horses through this beautiful work. Touch is a powerful tool with which to share our wonder of life. Many of my students have found that the ideas and techniques they experience in my courses have positively affected their lives outside the contact they have with horses. They experience life differently, they experience each other differently and they experience themselves differently. The respect, reverence and awe we feel as we share touch with horses spills over into daily life so that we live more sensitively toward ourselves and others. We become more conscious, more alive.

There is more to touching than skin to skin, or skin to hair contact. The touch that heals and teaches comes from a centered place within that we all possess. This part of us is our most natural self, the self that we know is closest to nature, free of judgements and even expectations. Sometimes people feel shocked the first time they experience the peace inside themselves that fosters healing in themselves and others. This is a place of dynamic relaxation, from where creativity can spring, this is also a place of pure love and joy. My first teacher of touch, Wataru Ohashi, has as his motto, 'Touch For Peace'.

Since my introduction to holistic medicine and Oriental healing arts in 1975, the scope and potential of these theories has fascinated me. I have also been fascinated by the modernization and expansion of simple practices that, in the desire of practitioners to become more mainstream, have had almost the opposite effect. The term 'New Age' may have divided Western medical practices from 'holistic' practices to the misfortune of those who would seek an alternative. Some holistic health practitioners have a 'them' and 'us' attitude toward the established, Descartes-rooted doctrine of rationalism.

WHY TOUCH FEELS SO GOOD

From the moment of conception, the fetus is surrounded by vertical pressure, that of the amniotic fluid. This surrounding support buoys, protects, and regulates body temperature. During the birth process, the pressure is increased as the baby moves through the birth canal, being alternately seized and thrust along until the ultimate shock of gravity forever changes everything. Life! Animal mothers then have the responsibility of physically stimulating the baby with licks and nudges, nibbles and immobile contact. It is a well-documented fact that any animals that lack contact with their mothers do not thrive. Living bodies naturally crave the contact and support that occurred during gestation.

THE IMPORTANCE OF HUMAN TO HUMAN CONTACT

When society became more 'high tech', humans began touching less and less. The hands-on healing modalities of many cultures gave way to machines and gadgets. Very often, the only physical contact a person has with his or her doctor is the handshake they exchange when they first meet, and sometimes not even that. Fortunately, we are again looking toward human contact for healing. It is well documented that newborns in intensive care units have a better survival rate when they are touched in a loving and healing way. Caregivers are learning specific techniques for these babies. Animals deprived of their mothers may not survive, even though they may be able to find food for themselves.

Most of us spent our early years in healthy close physical contact with our families. Then, at some point, children are discouraged from this contact, either by their parents, or by peer pressure. Several years go by until, hopefully, we find a mate. Some people never do. I have worked on people whose only physical contact was the one-hour shiatsu session they had with me. Isn't this sad?

I lived in London from 1970 to 1973. Most of this time was spent with an English family with four young children who are all parents now. We became very close and are still in touch. The middle daughter, Frances May, is one of my closest friends. Her son is now thirteen years old. I saw Danny when he was eleven, after ten years of not being in England. One of the first things he asked me was if I would give him some shiatsu. He paid close attention so he could work on his mother afterward. (He even asked me to teach him some techniques.) His mother told me that he enjoys giving massages to the family, and the back rub he gave me was terrific. He is a very wonderful lad, who was never told he was too big for snuggles.

During my early years in London, I would often go on outings with my adopted family. One day we were going off in the Land Rover, and some dust blew into five-year-old Dominic's eyes. They swelled shut and he panicked. I got him to calm down, as he became quite frantic from the pain and the fear from temporarily not being able to see. I did this by encouraging him to lie down, and I stroked his head, face, and eyes. He reminded me of this twenty years later. I had no training in touch at that time, but the human contact helped the frightened boy, whose tears washed away the grit from his eyes. He never forgot my soothing hands that day.

The partner stretching section in this book will get you into contact with another person's body in a healthy life-affirming way. It may even remind you that you are not getting enough attention yourself. Please seek out educated practitioners of touching modalities so you may better understand how your horse is feeling as you work on him. You will also learn a lot about your own body.

At the end of teaching each of my horse shiatsu courses, I present each student with a certificate and give them a hug. The first few times I taught in England, I noticed I was not always being hugged back with too much enthusiasm. I did not think it was because they did not enjoy the course but, rather, was reminded that, generally, the British are not an overly physically demonstrative society. For some reason though, for the last couple of years teaching in England and Scotland, I am getting some pretty terrific hugs. Maybe my teaching is improving.

Definitions

It is difficult to define the terms used to describe aspects of the oriental healing arts because many of these things defy logical explanations. With practice, however, comes more understanding and feel.

SHIATSU

Shiatsu is a Japanese word meaning finger pressure. **Shi** means 'finger' and **atsu** means 'pressure'. It is a sister modality to acupuncture and works along the same principles: that stimulation of certain points on and inside the body will have a positive effect on the body's ability to heal itself and restore health. Touch therapies have been used for thousands of years. Some of these therapies, such as shiatsu, have been refined to an art. Because of its status as an art, it has been creatively interpreted and further refined by many masters through the ages.

For five thousand years the Chinese have used acupuncture to prevent illness, maintain radiant good health and treat subtle manifestations of disease. The first acupuncture needles were probably sharp pieces of bone. It is said that the study of soldiers' injuries on the battlefield led to the discovery and development of acupuncture. The Chinese used *do in* and *anma* (which means press-rub) to stimulate points on the body of people and animals as a precursor to the insertion of needles on the same points. Do in is very similar to yoga while anma resembles western massage. These two techniques are the oldest forms of medical treatment in the Orient. Acupuncture needles can stimulate points just below the surface of the skin with shallow insertion, or go deep within the body, to stimulate points not accessible through touch. As time went by, acupuncture became enormously sophisticated and touching therapies such as acupressure became a companion therapy. (Acupressure is also called 'acupuncture without needles'.)

It is difficult to define the terms used to describe aspects of the oriental healing arts because many of these things defy logical explanations. With practice, however, comes more understanding and feel.

Touch therapies developed in the east, in China and India. In the twentieth century, the Japanese adopted acupressure and changed it in subtle ways to accommodate their lifestyle and needs and called it shiatsu. All styles of acupressure and massage are based on the principles of Chinese medicine. Swedish massage, although an entirely different focus from Asian bodywork therapies, originated in Asia and was introduced to the western world by a Swede.

The Japanese Ministry of Health and Welfare states 'Shiatsu therapy is a form of manipulation administered by the thumbs, fingers and palms, without the use of any instrument, mechanical or otherwise, to apply pressure to the human skin, correct internal malfunctioning, promote and maintain health and treat specific diseases'.

In Japan, anma is traditionally practiced by the blind for the purpose of comfort and pleasure. More recently authentic shiatsu came into being for the sole purpose of medical treatment. In *Zen Shiatsu*, Masunaga says that in both Zen and shiatsu we are dealing with something that cannot be explained rationally but that should be felt by the living body. In shiatsu, simply pressing will not reveal to you the life essence of what you are pressing. Without knowledge of oriental philosophy you will not be able to comprehend the meaning of life and will, therefore, administer shiatsu incorrectly.

Some practitioners practice mechanically, pressing a prescribed formula of points to cure disease. Other practitioners establish a rapport with the patient and can feel their life force and communicate with it to be successful in a long-term and beneficial way. This is the focus of this book. Masunaga states that in shiatsu the patient is master. We are trying to understand him or her physically, psychologically and spiritually.

The subtle energy or life force that flows through and around every living thing is called **chi** or **qi** in Chinese and **ki** in Japanese. Throughout this book, since my study of shiatsu has been through Japanese masters, I will refer to this energy as ki. Ki energy flows along meridians, vibrates through meridians to animate life. The balanced flow of this energy is both the cause and effect of good health. Since illness begins at a subtle level, an energetic level, prevention and treatment can begin with work at the energetic level in the body. For the practitioner of any bodywork therapy to be successful, they have the responsibility of being healthy. The practitioner must have an understanding and respect for the principles that formed the modality.

> Oriental medicine is not as rational as western medicine but if we respect the mysteries of life and make the patient aware of himself, disease will disappear and the patient will endeavour to get well on his own. By applying your hand on a point or tsubo and following the meridian lines with your fingers, you may feel the 'echo' of life. If you can receive and understand this sensation, disease will seem to disappear. Shizuto Masunaga

ENDORPHINS

Endorphins are neuropeptides (chemical messengers) within the brain with morphine-like properties. They suppress pain and regulate the body's natural response to stress. These natural analgesics are released during shiatsu and acupuncture, and are partially responsible for the relaxation response. Long-distance runners and swimmers experience a runner's or swimmer's 'high'. This is thought to be the result of the release of endorphins during prolonged physical exertion. This response is especially important for athletes who must recover quickly from injury. The release of endorphins may be the reason that injuries are not noticed until after the performance, during rest. There are more pathways sending touch sensation to the brain than those that send pain sensations.

KI ENERGY FLOWING THROUGH MERIDIANS

Ki is the subtle energy that is present in all life forms. The presence of ki signifies life, its absence, death. Recent research has detected that there are subtle energies moving through the body. Some sensitive practitioners can feel this energy. Anyone can learn to feel ki in another being. The unimpeded flow of ki through the body is related to a good healthy life.

Our bodies are composed of energy and information. Thoughts are energy. When you have a thought, there is a chemical reaction that is taking place. This thought may have a subtle or enormous effect on your body.

From ancient times the Chinese have considered the universe to comprise energy in various stages of vibration. Modern scholars of quantum physics are proving in their laboratories what the ancient Chinese have known for centuries, that ki energy is found in the tiniest particles that make up the form and substance of our universe.

Ki is everywhere, and in everything. It refers to energy in the widest sense. It has always been and will always be in space, time, matter, form and movement.

MERIDIANS

Meridians are channels that run throughout the body at various levels of depth. They carry ki to and from the internal organs. The subtle energy vibrating through the meridians has a higher frequency than matter. It is what maintains our vital life force.

The quality of energy perceived in these meridians can be divided into three **yang** qualities: sunlight yang, greater yang and lesser yang, and three **yin** qualities: absolute yin, greater yin and lesser yin. (A horse's forelegs each have three yin and three yang meridians and the hind legs also each have three different yin and yang meridians, thus there is a total of twelve meridians passing through the limbs.) The relationship between the organ and meridian exists in the functioning of the organ rather than the organ itself. Each meridian has a personality, expressing itself in balance and imbalance depending on its needs. Each has its own specific qualities of emotion, taste preference, smell relationships, time of day when most active or quiet, and expression at times of excitement and change.

In addition to the twelve 'regular' meridians there are eight additional channels which come into play in cases of emergency. These channels or pathways are reservoirs of Ki and are called vessels. We use two of these to treat certain forms of imbalance: the **Governing Vessel**, which is yang, and the **Conception Vessel**, which is yin; they are exceptional because they run down the center of the body, rather than bilaterally. The Governing Vessel influences all the yang meridians in the body and can be used to strengthen the yang energetic forces. The Conception Vessel influences all the yin meridians as well as the reproductive system.

The meridians are an interconnecting network of superficial and deep channels that flow throughout the body. Some run rather close to the surface of the body and some run deeply inside. The fourteen major meridians are superficial and have deep branches reaching to the major organs and connecting directly with each other. The pathways used by shiatsu practitioners lie one-eighth of an inch to four inches beneath the surface of the skin. It is along these pathways that **tsubos**, or acupuncture points, are located.

Tsubos, or classical acupuncture points, are places where ki accumulates along the meridians. In these areas, it is easier to tap into ki and manipulate it. Modern scientific investigation has shown that the tsubos are situated at places where there are particular physical features, for example: around joints, in the depressions between muscles, or where nerves run superficially. The electrical resistance of the skin at these points can be measured using electronic equipment and has been demonstrated to be lower than elsewhere on the body's surface.

The twelve primary meridians are partnered, or paired. Within each pair, one is yin, the other yang, functioning like sister and brother to keep harmony within and without. They are bilateral: each one has a mirror image of itself on the opposite side of the body. Ten of these primary meridians are organ related, represent the function of major organs of the body and are named after the body's organs:

Lung (yin) and **Large Intestine** (yang) Lu and LI
Spleen (yin) and **Stomach** (yang) Sp and St
Heart (yin) and **Small Intestine** (yang) Ht and SI
Kidney (yin) and **Bladder** (yang) K and Bl
Liver (yin) and **Gall Bladder** (yang) Li and GB

The yin organ meridians relate to solid organs, the yang organ meridians relate to hollow organs. The yin meridians run along the inside of the limbs, and the yang meridians run along the outside.

In addition to these ten organ-related meridians are the **Heart Constrictor** Meridian, (yin, HC) also called Pericardium or Circulation Sex, and the **Triple Heater** Meridian, (yang TH) also called Triple Warmer. The Heart Constrictor represents the system of veins and arteries which the Chinese recognize as a separate organ. This meridian also functions as a protector of the Heart Meridian, which is sensitive and vulnerable. It protects against physical imbalances as well as emotional bumps and bruises of everyday life. It governs the ease and flow of sexual activity and function. The Triple Heater Meridian relates to the lymphatic system and governs the function of thermal regulation throughout the body. The word 'triple' refers to the upper, middle, and lower burning spaces in the body, as described in ancient Chinese texts. The upper burning space represents the organs of respiration, the middle burning space represents the organs of digestion, and the lower burning space represents the organs of elimination.

The meridians refer not only to the function of the organ, but to an entire realm of qualities which are necessary for the harmonious functioning of the **bodymindspirit**. (*See* Meridian Characteristics.)

In a healthy individual, the energy in these meridians flows freely in a balanced state. When abnormal functioning of the internal organs or abnormal external stimulation occur, energy stagnates, becomes excessive, or depleted in the meridians. This is the precursor to disease and first occurs on a subtle, or energetic, level. For the body to recover health, the energy in these channels must be stimulated, or sedated, then released to become normalized. The release of energy can be to other meridians, or out of the body.

Experienced practitioners are able to feel this unbalanced energy and work with it to help restore homeostasis. Anyone can learn to work with energy if properly taught.

BODYMINDSPIRIT

In Oriental medicine, the physical, mental and spiritual aspects of an individual are treated as a whole, not as separate entities. We are integrated beings; each of the components of body, mind and spirit are affected by the others and become one: bodymindspirit.

YIN AND YANG

Ki is separated into different qualities or forces that interact. Chinese scholars developed the theory of yin and yang to describe and make sense of the real world. Broad and all-encompassing, the yin/yang theory can be used to help us understand life around us, and life within us. The possibilities of application are endless: how we act and react, our likes and dislikes, cravings etc. On a universal level, yin and yang help us understand the ebb and flow of tides, the obvious and subtle life force that animates, political and social trends and even natural disasters.

The circle that is the symbol of yin and yang shows us that within every yin quality there is an aspect of yang, and vice versa. The circle symbolizes the wholeness and infinity of ki, having neither beginning nor ending. There is a curved line separating the two halves of the circle, signifying movement of energy, and the flow of yin into yang and yang into yin. Within each portion is a dot representing the other. This dot shows us that there are no absolutes and that everything contains the seeds of its opposite within it. There is no hot without cold, no up without down and no wet without dry. The two halves are in equal proportion, illustrating a dynamic balance.

The original meanings of yin and yang were 'the shady side of a hill' and 'the sunny side of a hill' respectively.

Yin and yang represent the duality of nature. The Chinese divided life into forces which support and destroy each other, in a natural sequence of things. This concept is at the root of the philosophy of traditional Chinese medicine. Yin and yang coexist with each other and within each other. Yin and yang have their natural cycles of interplay, for example, the sun is yang, an energy that is strong and obvious, the moon, yin, gives more subtle energy. During the times of dawn and dusk, there is an obvious interplay of yin and yang, not quite night, but not quite day. There are forces of yin and yang in living bodies controlling obvious and subtle functions, for example, the lungs, a yin organ, give off waste material in the form of gasses that cannot be seen; the large intestine, a yang organ, eliminates body waste that is visible. In Chinese medicine, these two organs support each other in the world of yin and yang.

Male and female energies are an obvious example of the yin/yang theory. Male energy (yang) is said to be more obvious, expanded, pushing and active, while female energy (yin) is more subtle, receptive, quiet and sensitive.

When yin and yang energies become unbalanced, **kyo** and **jitsu** occur. Many problems begin with tiredness. One of my early teachers said the best advice the practitioner can give the patient is to rest. Rest restores our energy and helps us avoid problems.

For example, you and your horse have been busy training and preparing for an important event. You are so driven (yang energy) to succeed that you take no time for your own rest and proper nutrition. Your nervous energy has transferred to your usually calm horse who is restless even when at rest. While training intensely (yang activity) you are not taking time to focus on giving shiatsu to him (yin activity), or receiving any yourself. You realize that you are catching a cold and you and your horse are not accomplishing too much. You give him a last minute shiatsu session to increase his energy (using up your own depleted energy). You release his reserves of energy that he should be using for self-restoration (yin) and he burns if off during the event (yang). Resolving the symptom has not resolved the problem. He takes longer to recover his energy because he is using reserves of energy, and possibly gets hurt during the show from a pulled muscle (yin). This muscle pull takes longer to recover because his body is too exhausted and depleted to contract the expanded muscle injury. Your cold keeps getting worse and now you are depressed (yin) because you cannot ride your horse. By keeping adequate balance throughout this process, all these compounded problems could have been avoided. The tiredness is the kyo, characterized by excessive yang activity without the balance of yin.

The posterior part of the body is yang while the anterior part is yin. It is said that the yang is the more protective, the yin is protected. The yang parts of the body are exposed to the energy of the sun (yang). The skin, hair, and musculature of the yang parts of the body are more visible. The yang is also tougher than the yin. In treating the body, we can touch the yang portions of the body with stronger pressure. It can take more stimulation. The yin parts, hidden and protected, have less hair, are softer and more delicate, and need to be treated with more gentleness.

KYO AND JITSU

Kyo and jitsu describe the energy (ki) imbalances or distortions within the meridian lines. Somewhat similar to the concepts of yin and yang, kyo is the condition of depleted energy, which is more hypo, and jitsu is the condition of excessive energy, which is more hyper. Kyo is the cause and jitsu is the result. The result is the symptom (jitsu) or the physical manifestation of the problem.

Masunaga illustrates this by asking us to think of a perfectly round ball representing a healthy person. Now think of a distorted ball with indentations and protrusions marring its circumference. The indentations, which are hollow and below the surface, are the areas of kyo, the protrusions are jitsu. The jitsu areas are easier to spot because they protrude from the surface and are obvious. It is more difficult to detect the kyo areas because they are subtle. The kyo is the cause of the problem, the jitsu the result. If the practitioner only treats the jitsu, as in some types of bodywork therapy, to sedate the overabundant energy, the patient may feel better, but only temporarily, as the cause of the problem, the kyo, is still waiting to be addressed.

The quality of kyo feels empty, hollow, cold or cool, inactive and receptive. It is a void, lacking in energy. Upon palpation, you may find your hand feels pulled in and held. It may also feel stiff and resistant, possibly as a defence mechanism, after a time. If this is the case, it feels as if there is jitsu hiding kyo. Upon palpation, the stiffness may suddenly release, revealing the kyo hidden beneath. Kyo requires patient holding, because it takes time for healing warmth to reach deep inside to nurture, strengthen and to normalize the area. This holding is called **tonification.** In many cases, simply using tonification for the kyo will normalize the jitsu. As depleted energy is restored – the energy has come from somewhere else in the body, often the jitsu – thus balance has been restored.

> Since kyo is fundamental to any disease, it must be tonified in order to cure the disease. Shizuto Masunaga.

In classic Chinese medical books this concept of unbalanced kyo and jitsu is known as **jyaki**, the condition of energy distortion.

Working slowly and using palm pressure is typically tonifying. However, an entire session of slow, methodical techniques of long holding may overly relax the patient, causing the feeling of excessive tiredness. The areas to be tonified are only the most kyo. If the entire body is kyo, the practitioner must determine the most kyo, and not overwork the individual.

The quality of jitsu feels active, warm or hot, stiff, or hard and tight. The jitsu area may reject your touch because of the excessive energy there, and the lack of any need for receiving further energy. This blocked energy may have pooled in an area due to injury or habit, and needs to be addressed in a stronger way than the kyo, which requires patient nurturing. The techniques for dealing with jitsu are pressure of shorter duration, sharper penetration and working in the opposite direction of energy flow in the meridian line the jitsu is in. Sometimes strong manipulation techniques are used, such as overstretching, percussion and certain chiropractic techniques. The techniques used in treating jitsu are called **sedation**.

Using pointed elbows and thumbs is appropriate for sedation, although elbows and thumbs can be used in a tonifying way.

Meridian Work

Although the traditional theory of Chinese acupuncture states that energy flows in specific directions along meridians, and that you should work within the direction of energy flow to bring energy to the meridian (tonify) and in the opposite direction to remove energy (sedate), I work everything away from the center of the body, in the style of the late Master Shizuto Masunaga. His theory is that all energy emanates outward from the center of the body, and that the way we touch and communicate with the meridian determines whether we are achieving tonification or sedation.

There are many ways you can work along meridian lines and get positive results. The most simple and basic way is to work rhythmically without varying your pressure and speed, going along at medium speed and pressure. If you want to accomplish something however, I suggest you use the Meridian Characteristics section (*see* pages 166–77) to determine which meridians you will work on. Working them all is too time consuming and does not accomplish much apart from sending too many messages to the body. Choose two or three to work on. The Bladder Meridian is always a good choice for one of them, unless the horse's back is so sore and painful you are unable to. You may base your choice on either psychological or physical characteristics, or a combination of both.

The way you touch the horse will be determined by many factors. You should first determine if he is a yin or yang type horse (*see* pages 230 and 231). Try to match the energy of each horse you work on. If he is highly strung, work more quickly in the beginning of the session, gradually slowing down as he becomes relaxed, which is very important for this type of horse. If working on a quiet, unexcitable or uninterested horse, work slowly at first and pick up your speed to enliven him a little.

If working on a horse in a weak or tired condition, or a very yin type, or one who has just recovered from illness, work slowly along the meridian, staying at least ten seconds in each location. Your pressure will be gentle but deep, or very light, depending on his reaction to your touch, and also the reaction to the points you use on the meridian. You will concentrate on finding the areas that feel most depleted (kyo) and stay in these areas until you feel some response.

A kyo point usually feels like an indentation under the skin, or a hollow spot. You may feel very little in the way of circulation or energy flow. The response we are hoping for is a filling-up feeling of the empty kyo places. As soon as you feel some reaction under your palm, fingertips, or thumb, move on to the next point. If you do not feel any response after about fifteen seconds, move on to the next point. If you do feel a response (increased circulation, warmth, tingling, or an actual filling up of the hollow area), stay a second or two longer, then move on to the next point. If you come to a jitsu area (hard, tight, hot, stiff or reactive, or all of these) just make a note of its location and pass it by. The second time you work on the meridian, you may not find it, as the stagnant unreleased energy may have released. The horse will feel kyo and jitsu points as distinctly different from each other. Usually he will accept pressure in the kyo areas because, although they may be a bit sensitive, it is a comfortable satisfying feeling to be touched there. Ohashi refers to this feeling as 'comfortable pain'. The area may not be sensitive at all, rather almost numb, as no energy is moving there. A jitsu point or area is usually sore, and he will not appreciate strong pressure there. Ohashi calls this 'nasty pain'.

If working on a horse who is very energetic, in blooming health, full of himself, in regular work, and is a yang type, you should work specifically and firmly, even though your demeanour will of course be gentle. He will not appreciate any vacillation on your part. You must be very focused in order not to lose his attention.

WHY WORK ON MERIDIANS?

You may be able to accomplish a lot without working on a single meridian line but, for the results to be lasting, it is important to reinforce your physical movement techniques with energy work. Working on meridians can help the body adjust itself in certain cases of misalignment. This is because when energy is where it is supposed to be in a balanced way, the body is able to adjust itself. In situations where there is an organ imbalance that is affecting energy flow, that in turn may be causing pain that affects movement; meridian work, along with your vet's advice, will help the body to right itself. Meridian work reinforces the purely physical work you do with your horse during shiatsu. We are working with energy in any case, but working on meridians and points gives this work the refinement that makes it so versatile. Meridian work establishes wholeness and the continuation of healing after the session has ended.

Preparing Yourself

As a practitioner of shiatsu with horses, I endeavor to bring to all my activities the focus I need to have to practice and teach this work effectively. If I give 100 per cent of my concentration, effort and focus to my work and then go home and sloppily wash the dishes or cut the grass without paying attention to the potential for excellence in the task, I am not giving myself the opportunity to grow in all my tasks. Eventually, my work may suffer because of this generally uncaring attitude in my life. Now, striving to be mindful of my work throughout my life is not an easy task for me; I believe my attitude leans towards laziness, and I have the tendency to take the easy way out. It is, therefore, easy for me to believe that we teach what we most need to learn; we teach something because it is a way for us to develop ourselves – and to move closer to realizing our own potential – as well as helping and guiding the development of others.

With this in mind, I try to create opportunities for myself throughout the day to be mindful of and fully present in my tasks. If I am talking to someone and I am in a hurry to go to my next appointment, I must be fully present with that person, and as I drive to the next appointment, I focus on my driving, and when I arrive, my attention becomes focused on the task and individuals I am with, not the problems at the place I have just left. Try this sometime when you have a busy day. Try to be with each situation and in the present.

PREPARING THE HEALER WITHIN

In a perfect world we would all be centered all the time. However, it is particularly important to be strongly centered before and during shiatsu with horses for effectiveness and safety. Horses are enormously sensitive and will often reflect our mental state. When working with your horse, doing shiatsu or anything else, be in the moment, not preoccupied. Let go of your thoughts, expectations, ego and worries, and be here now. Whatever you need to do to center yourself, find something that resonates comfortably within. It may be a meditation, visualization, a mantra, or prayer. My own procedure varies from time to time. When traveling to a horse, a mile from my destination I begin to focus on the horse. I turn off the music, focus on breathing low in my abdomen and relaxing my body. I empty my mind and bring my attention to the horse. (Of course I am also concentrating on the road.)

I may get a picture of the horse, complete with color and body type. I particularly notice if one area stands out in my mind's eye. Most of the time this is where the problem is (I usually do not ask the owner too many questions before I see the horse to avoid preconceived ideas and expectations unless it is an emergency). I extend my energy to the horse and let him or her know that I am on my way to help. I send loving thoughts of admiration and acceptance. Upon arrival I ask the horse if I may enter the stall. If the feeling is yes, I enter quietly and respectfully. I kneel or squat in the corner and pray that I may be used to the best advantage in this moment. I open my heart to this perfect expression of life as a partner in healing, and a nonjudgmental listener. I greet and affirm the intelligence, sensitivity, grace, strength and beauty of the perfect being before me. I am at peace.

HEALTH AND THE FOOD WE EAT

Another important aspect of the practitioner of a healing art is to be able to maintain the health and clarity of your own body. To be a channel for the healing power of the universe to come through, the channel must be clear. Therefore, I feel it is extremely important to be in as healthy and strong a condition as possible. Each person needs to find the diet that is most beneficial to them and this may change as the person changes and when life stresses, environment and seasons change. Remember that all dietary changes should be made gradually and gently.

Make a list of everything you eat for one week. If there is anything that contains a list of ingredients, especially things you are unable to pronounce, it probably is not good for you. Try to eat things in their most fresh condition, without overcooking or adding unnecessary extras. Eat only a minimum of animal protein if you must eat any at all. Eat grains, not processed in cereals but cooked in water. Avoid junk food, fast food and sweets as much as possible. Keep alcohol consumption to a minimum and remember that caffeine takes your energy, it does not give it to you. Drink lots of fresh water. If your body, which has the potential to become like a tuning fork for healing, has clarity, your mind will become focused more easily and you will be energized by your work rather than fatigued by it.

This is not to say that we must live in a bubble and not partake of the many interesting tastes and smells and sensations that our world has to offer. I have known strict vegetarians who make those around them uncomfortable by their fanaticism, especially in restaurants. It is unfair (and poor manners) to impose such restrictions on our companions. Rather, set a quiet, elegant example by what you do and when others are ready to make their own changes, they will do so, in their own good time.

Also, if you are ready to make some positive lifestyle changes yourself, please do so gently. Many people have observed that they become ill when changing their diets and that a healthy diet does not work for them. Any sudden change will affect the body's chemistry drastically and, as it detoxifies, old illnesses may resurface, aches and pains will come out, and even skin changes may occur.

In the years since 1983 during which I have been working with horses and their humans, I have noticed that many people take better care of all their animals than they do of themselves. I have listened as they discuss the latest research of the supplements that they carefully measure and add to the best feed they can afford to buy (and some they cannot afford). I have watched as they give their horses time to rest when an injury that could affect their future occurs. I have happily looked on as they groom their lovely and beloved horses, all the while speaking sweetly and bestowing kisses generously. These same caring people then feed themselves food with such minor nutritious value (and even dangerous ingredients) that it makes me wonder how they have the energy to stay on a horse's back.

It is not just what we eat but how we manage a meal that is important. Try to avoid mealtime stress. This would include upsetting conversations, watching the news and reading the newspaper. Keep your taking-in process focused only on food rather than information.

Premeal Meditation

Before you lift an eating utensil, close your eyes, or look at your food, and take a deep breath. As you exhale slowly, let all thoughts go and focus on your food. Take a moment to be grateful to all those who helped in supplying this meal for you. Then, ask that this food sustains you in your tasks and contributes to the health and wellbeing of your body, mind and spirit. Take your first bite and really chew it well, to allow your saliva to begin the breaking-down process before you swallow. Try to feel how your body is reacting to this first bite, then send it down. Eat slowly so that you do not overtax your stomach; you will get much more benefit from your food as your intestines are able to absorb nutrients from your meal, rather than just working to digest and eliminate. Take the time to feel the effect of your food on your body.

One of my early teachers said that what we take in is not as important as how well we eliminate. This man is blessed with a strong constitution and can eat anything. He also said the best taste was fresh water. He was dipping huge fresh strawberries in melted chocolate at the time, followed by an espresso coffee and a European cigarette. Evaluate your capabilities and support them.

Associate yourself with people who uplift your spirit, teach you and learn from you as well. Spend time with children, acting in a childlike manner with them. Be generous with your smiles. Spend as much time appreciating nature as you can. Please be happy!

SELF-SHIATSU ADVICE

Work slowly and breathe deeply but comfortably. If any points are sensitive or painful, hold them a bit longer, or increase or decrease your pressure. It may feel good to do self-shiatsu before or after doing meridian stretches. You may wish to exhale as you press each point and inhale as you move into the next one. Do these techniques with full attention on your body and what it may be communicating to you. Self-shiatsu is very helpful if you feel a cold coming on, or are ill and cannot leave the house. It will keep energy going, improve your circulation and relax your body.

Self-shiatsu

Arms

Sit as shown, with your buttocks between your heels, or with crossed legs. Grasp your upper arm and squeeze gently, working your way from your upper arm to your elbow *(left and center)*. You may work several places along the way, holding each location for from three to ten seconds, or whatever feels comfortable. Repeat on the other arm. To work the forearm, place it on the floor in front of you and, with the other arm, lean rather than press into it, working from the elbow toward the wrist *(right, top and bottom)*. Work several locations, with comfortable pressure. Repeat on the other arm, then sit up and take a moment to feel the relaxing, energizing effects.

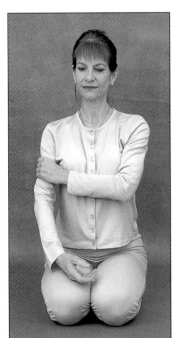
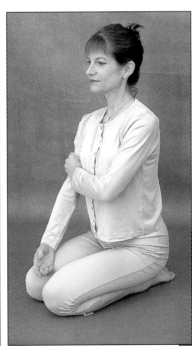
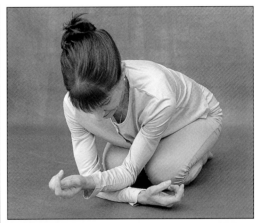
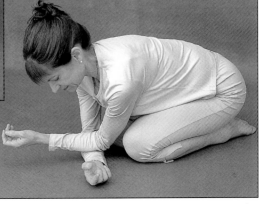

Neck

Clasp your hands and place the heels of your hands on the large muscles at the back of your neck, then, bring your elbows toward each other, creating pressure on the muscles, and stretch your neck forward. Start at the top of your neck and proceed to its base, touching two or three locations along the way. Begin each sequence with your head up and your elbows out to the side, as shown in the first photo.

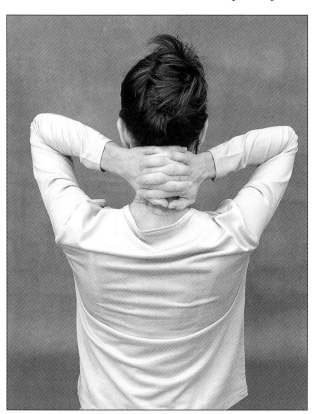
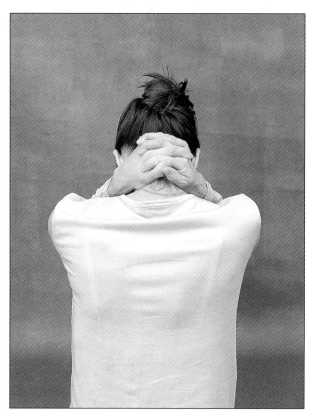

Shoulders

Place your fingertips on the muscle on top of your shoulder and hold your elbow with the other hand. Pull your elbow downward, creating the fingertip pressure in your shoulder *(opposite, top left)*. (Working in this manner helps avoid tension in the shoulder of the working hand.) Once you are pressing the muscle in your shoulder with firm pressure, hold it and stretch your neck gently toward the other shoulder and slightly forward *(opposite, top center)*. Hold this position for several seconds or whatever feels comfortable. Then, lift your head up, push your elbow so that your fingertips reach farther down behind your shoulder, press them into the muscle by pulling your elbow downward, and stretch your neck forward and slightly to the side. Repeat this technique until you have worked several points, from the top of your shoulder to about a quarter of the way down your back if possible. Repeat on the other side, then take a moment to observe the comfortable feeling in your shoulders.

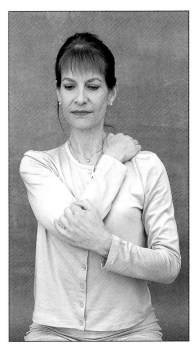
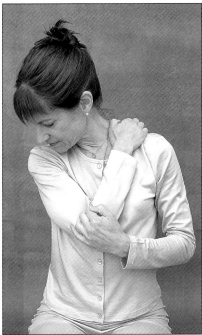
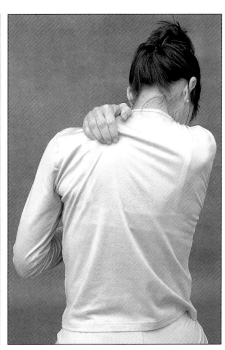

Back

Sit as shown or with your legs crossed. Place your thumbs in the large muscles next to your spine, as high as you can without tensing your shoulders *(below, left and right)*. When the thumbs are firmly in position, lean your body rearward to create a bit more pressure. Hold for several seconds. Place the thumbs in the next location, about an inch down, and repeat. Work all the way down your back in this way, then lean forward to stretch the muscles.

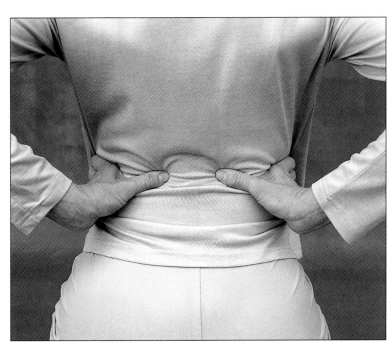
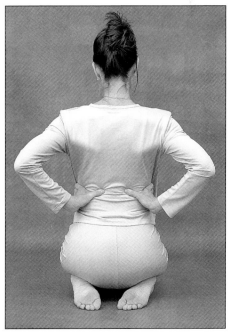

Legs and feet, sitting

Sit as shown, and place your elbows on top of and slightly to the sides of your thighs. Walk them down toward your knees, left, right, left, right, with comfortable pressure. *(Top left.)* Then, place your fingertips slightly under your calves, to the outside of the shinbone, pressing upward firmly. Lean to the right slightly, creating pressure, then to the left. Move your fingers down toward your ankles, alternating as you go. *(Top right.)* Then, reach around and place your knuckles on the soles of your feet, leaning into one, then the other, working on the entire sole of your foot. *(Bottom.)*

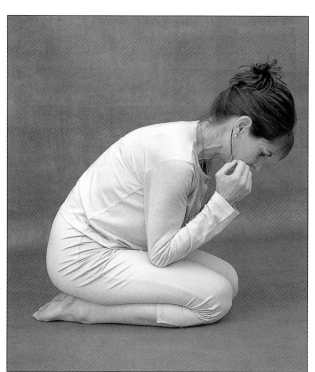

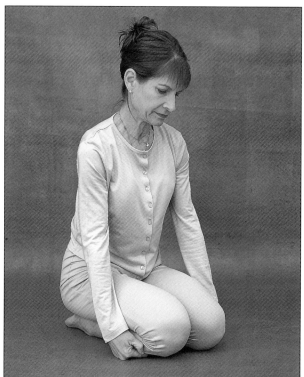

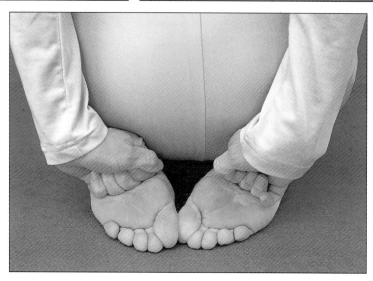

Legs in supine position

Cross your legs so that the heel of your foot is against the outside of your thigh, as high up toward your hip as possible (you may use your hand to help you get it up there). Press your heel into your leg and your leg into your heel, and hold for a few seconds. Work in increments from the top of your thigh toward your knee, then continue down your leg toward your ankle. Uncross your legs and repeat on the other leg. *(Top, left and right.)* Then, open one leg outward on the floor with your knee bent. Starting at the ankle, walk your heel up your calf and thigh in small increments, pressing down gently but firmly and holding each location for a few seconds. *(Bottom, left and right.)* Repeat on the other leg. Then, rest in a comfortable position for a few minutes at least and observe the pleasant sensations in your body.

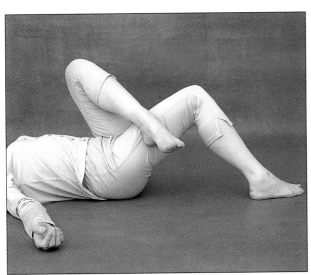
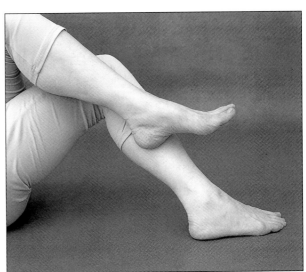

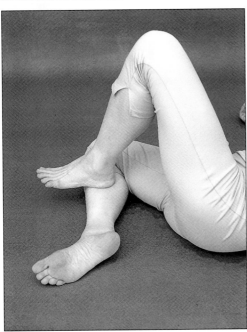
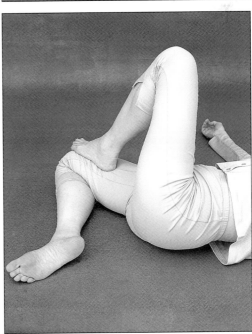

Meridian Stretches

None of these exercises should cause pain. The sensation of gentle stretching feels good. Always breathe deeply and slowly. If any dizziness occurs, gradually come out of the stretch and rest. Never compete with yourself and try to do more than your intuition tells you. Be especially careful if you suffer from chronic back pain or have ever dislocated your shoulders. Never bounce, rather use your slow, even breathing to take you further into the stretches as you become proficient. Always take a moment to rest and observe your body after each stretch. Note the stretch in terms of where you feel your energy flowing through your body or where it may feel blocked. Concentrate on relaxing and releasing during all these movements, and enjoy!

After completing the series of stretches, always rest for a moment, preferably lying on the floor in a comfortable position, such as on your back with your knees bent.

LARGE INTESTINE AND LUNG MERIDIANS

Hook your thumbs behind your back, and point your index fingers. (Lung Meridian ends in the thumbs and Large Intestine Meridian begins in the index fingers.) Stand with your feet hip width apart,

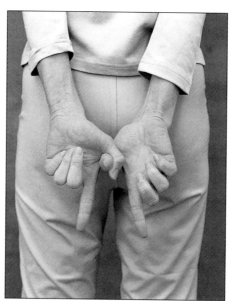
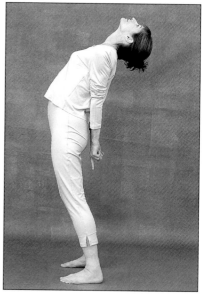

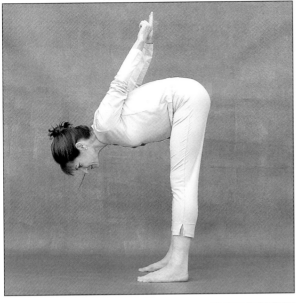
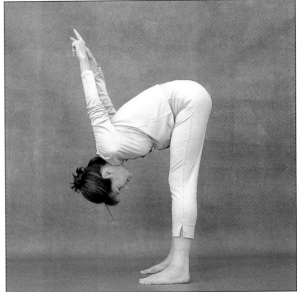
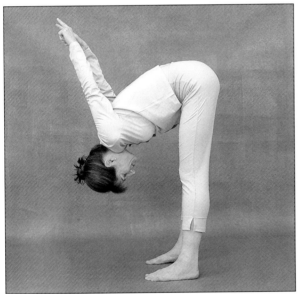
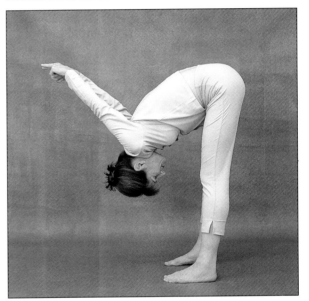

and the outside edges of your feet parallel. You may feel as if your toes are turned slightly inward. Keep your knees soft throughout this exercise. Take a deep breath in and lean slightly rearward by pressing your abdomen forward, creating a gentle arch in your back. Breathe out as you bend slowly forward from your hips. Allow your shoulders to release and your hands to rise upward. During the next three or four breathes, go further into the stretch, allowing your shoulders to relax and release as your head moves closer to your knees. Your neck should be relaxed so that you feel gravity stretching your neck. If you are not able to breathe deeply, perhaps you are stretching too much and should rise back up slightly. Come out of the stretch on an inhalation, slowly, reverse the position of the thumbs and repeat the sequence.

BLADDER AND KIDNEY MERIDIANS

Sit with your legs stretched in front of you, hip width apart. Flex your feet until you feel the stretch in your calves. Sit up very straight, lifting slightly out of your hips if possible. Now, clasp your hands, and invert the clasp, pressing your palms toward the ceiling, as you breathe in. Really reach up out of your hips. Next, as you slowly exhale, bend forward and stretch your palms toward the wall in front of you. This will keep you from compressing the abdominal area. Keep your arms alongside your ears. With each exhalation, stretch a tiny bit further forward (about three or four breaths all together). On the last inhalation, rise up, palms facing the ceiling, lifting out of the hips. Then release the hands, stretching the arms outward, and down to your sides. Take a moment to observe your body for signals of tightness. You may feel some sensation in the backs of the legs and knees, lower back, or shoulders.

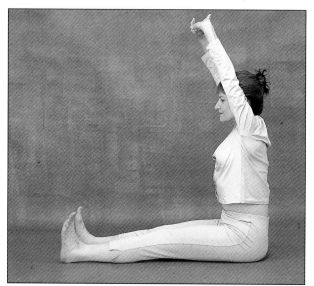
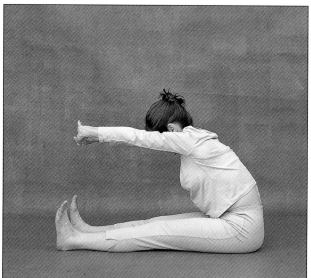
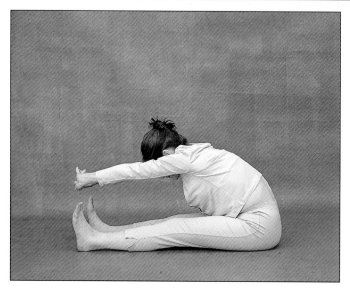

GALL BLADDER AND LIVER MERIDIANS

Stretch your legs outward, with your feet flexed and your knees facing upward. Clasp your hands, invert the clasp, take a deep breath in, and lift your body upward out of your hips. *(Top left.)* Turn toward your right leg, and begin to stretch your body to your left side. *(Top right and bottom left.)* Stop stretching as you breathe in, and stretch further on the exhalation. The direction of the stretch is beyond your foot so you do not collapse the left side of your body. The purpose is to lengthen both sides of your body. Take about three or four breaths to attain your maximum stretch. Try to keep your elbow to the inside of your knee, and your face forward. Sit up on your next inhalation, lifting out of your hips, turn to the left, and repeat the stretch to the right, extending toward and past your foot. *(Bottom right.)* To come out of this position, place your hands on the floor behind you, lift your hips, pull your body slightly back and bring your legs together, then shake them out.

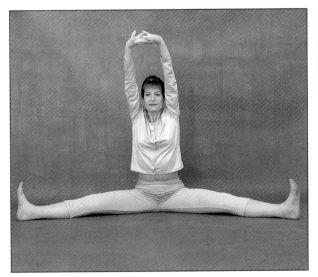
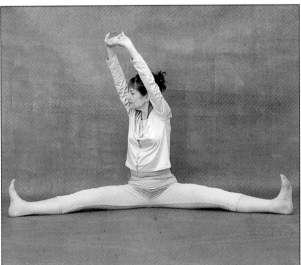
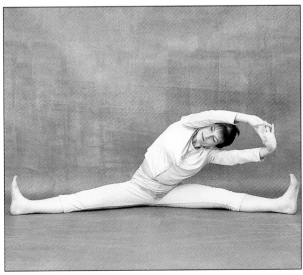
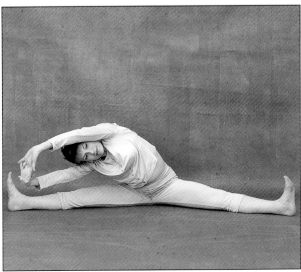

SMALL INTESTINE AND HEART MERIDIANS

Sit up very straight with the soles of your feet together and your hands clasped around them. Your arms should be straight. Take a deep breath in, and on the exhalation begin to stretch your body forward, stretching your elbows outward, and keeping your knees as close to the floor as possible. Move your body further forward on each of three or four breaths all together, until your elbows are close to the floor. Sit back up on the inhalation and stretch your back upward for one more breath. Extend your legs in front of you and shake them out.

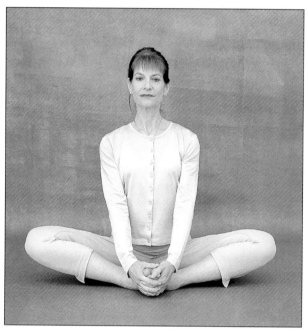
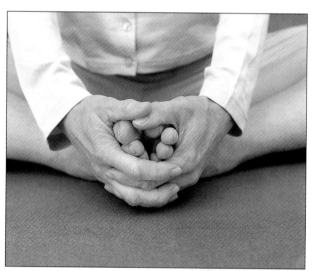
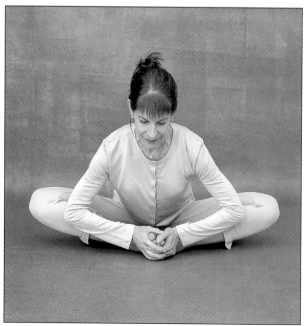
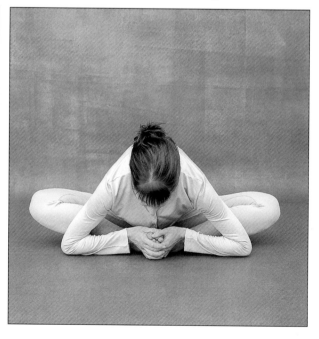

TRIPLE HEATER AND HEART CONSTRICTOR MERIDIANS

Cross your legs, then cross your arms and place your hands over your knees. Take a deep breath in and on the exhalation, bend your body forward until your elbows touch the floor. This may be done in one breath. Stay in this position for three or four breaths, then sit up on the inhalation. Recross your legs and your arms, reversing the position of each, and repeat the stretch.

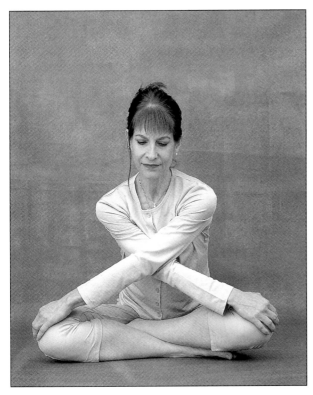

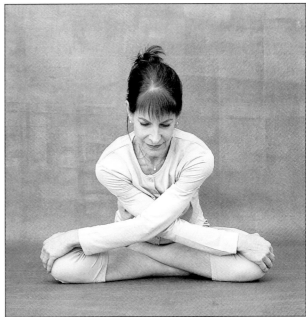

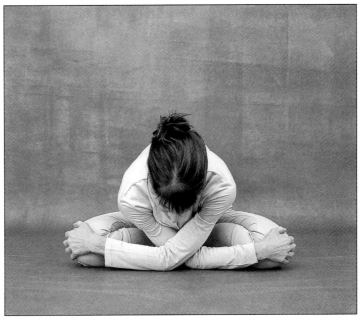

STOMACH AND SPLEEN MERIDIANS

Sit between your heels with your knees about hip width apart. Place your palms on the floor just behind your feet. Take a deep breath in and on the exhalation, bend the elbows to the floor. If your knees begin to pop up off the floor, stay in a position with your elbows only slightly bent. If you are completely comfortable in this position, with your knees firmly on the floor, on the next exhalation, lower your back the rest of the way to the floor, clasp your hands, invert the clasp and stretch your palms toward the wall behind you. Try to keep your back as close to the floor as possible. To come out of the stretch, reverse the sequence. First, place your forearms on the floor, then your palms. Lean completely forward at the end and lightly tap your lower back with your hands.

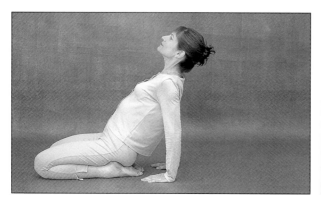
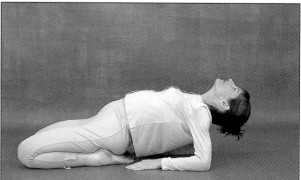

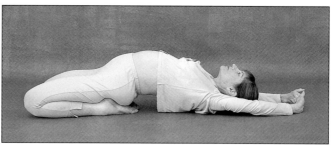

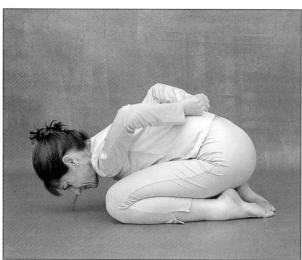
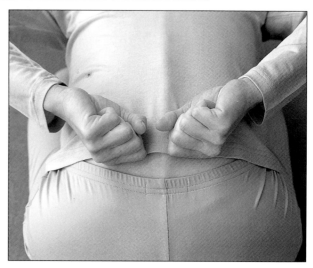

Partner Stretching

Stretching by yourself is important and can even be used as a moving meditation. Stretching with a partner is fun and educational for both of you. As the receiver of assisted stretching, you become increasingly aware of your body and its possibilities. While being stretched, it is important that you remember the stretching is just for you and you do not have to do more to please or impress the person helping you to stretch. Also, you are not in competition with each other. Each of you has individual needs, abilities and a history of stresses, strains and injuries that have influenced your present condition.

While you are being stretched, keep your attention on your body and breathing. You should be able to breathe deeply, smoothly and evenly as you are stretching. Always move into the stretch on an exhalation. This will help your muscles to relax and release.

The helper may need to remind you to breath more deeply and audibly as you are stretching. The helper should also be verbally encouraging during the stretches, and frequently ask you if you are comfortable, want to go further, or are feeling overstretched. Be aware of your body and what it is saying to you as you go into, come out of, and rest after each exercise. Notice how you feel if you are being understretched and need to be helped to go further. Notice how you feel if you are being overstretched and begin to feel pain or panicky. Your breathing will immediately change, becoming irregular and shallow. Most of all, be aware of how satisfying it is to be assisted just enough by your partner. This will feel comfortable and safe.

It is important to notice all these things by yourself, as they will help you to understand how your horse is feeling as you stretch him. The assisted stretches will help you become a more confident helper to your horse. As you begin to practice the stretching exercises on your horse, be aware of his breathing, or have someone listen to his breathing and tell you what is happening as you stretch him. Feel his reaction as you felt your own during the assisted stretches. Become one with him.

When it is your turn to help stretch your partner, ask for verbal feedback. Keep in contact with your partner by asking some questions as you proceed into the stretch, such as 'Are you comfortable?', or 'Would you like to try to stretch further?', or 'Tell me when you are at your comfortable maximum stretch'. With each answer, you will learn through your hands and in your body what your partner is feeling. In the photos notice that I am using my body to take my partner with me rather than pushing her with my hands. I am also breathing with her, to be more in contact with what she is experiencing. This will help you to be confident as you are learning to stretch your horse. As the helper, you will know what they are experiencing during an insufficient stretch, during too much of a stretch, and the perfect amount of stretch. Your instincts will improve so that you know exactly how long to hold a stretch. Usually about five seconds maximum works well, although in some cases you may wish to shorten or lengthen the time slightly.

Please enjoy this time with your human partner, and practice the partner stretches with several different people, possibly even before you work on your horse.

PARTNER STRETCHING ADVICE

Learn the stretches well individually before you attempt them with a partner. This will allow you to explore the subtleties of each stretch. It will also enable you to give very clear instructions to your partner about form and breathing. When teaching these stretches to another person, always remind them to breathe deeply, do not force any of the movements, and enjoy the sensations. Also, take a minute or two to observe the benefits of each stretch upon its completion before going on to the next position. Never compete with each other as each body has its own unique ability to move. As with the meridian stretches, rest for a moment after completing these stretches, preferably lying on the floor in a comfortable position, such as on your back with your knees bent.

Lung and Large Intestine Meridians

Observe your partner as she prepares for the stretch. Direct her to breathe in as she leans back, and breathe out as she begins to lean forward. Observe her back for any area of tension as she proceeds to maximum forward stretch position. An area may appear tight, or full, or tense. Trust your instincts, and place one hand over this area, which will bring awareness to your partner's body and facilitate release. Your other hand contacts her behind both wrists. She will take another deep breath and upon the exhalation, relax more into the stretch. As she slowly exhales, ask if she is in her maximum stretch position. If so, on the next exhalation, lean your body gradually toward her, exerting slight pressure on her back and equal pressure on each wrist. This is careful and subtle, not at all forced. You are helping your partner reach a maximum stretch and to discover a new maximum. She may stay in the stretched position for two or three breaths. Upon each inhalation, release pressure from your hands, on exhalation re-establish your pressure. On the last inhalation, she will begin to straighten up. Keep your hands on her as she stands, as the increased oxygenation may cause slight dizziness. Note that throughout this sequence her knees must not be locked but soft.

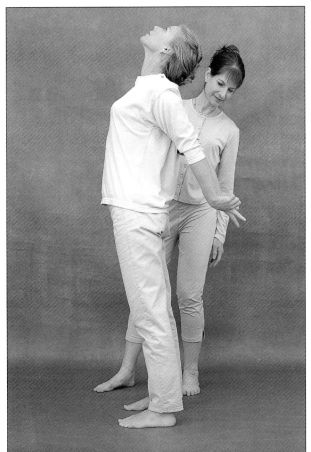
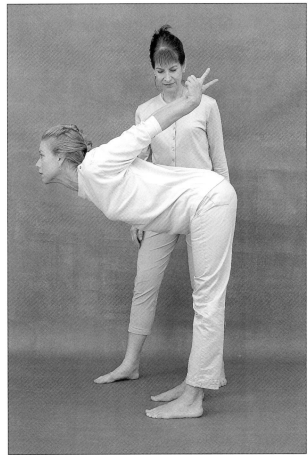

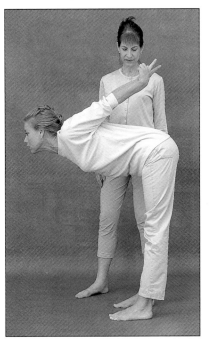
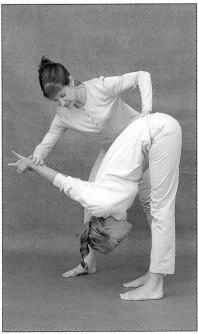
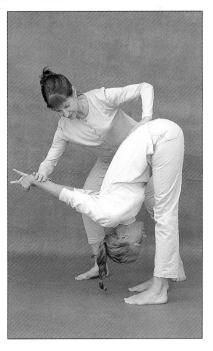

Bladder and Kidney Meridians

Your partner will assume the beginning posture, feet flexed, hands clasped and inverted. Upon her first inhalation, lift her slightly upward by holding her upper ribcage from the sides and raising your body slightly and taking her with you. Continue to support her as she progresses to full stretch forward position, taking about three exhalations to get there. With her next exhalation, help her stretch forward by leaning your body toward the wall in front of you, not downward. For the next two or three exhalations, help her stretch, releasing pressure but not hand contact as she inhales. On the last inhalation she comes back up, you lift her slightly upward again, and release contact.

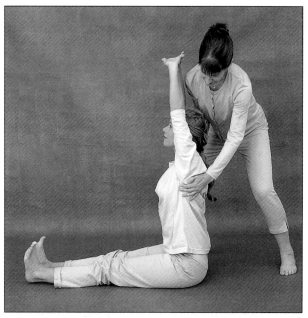
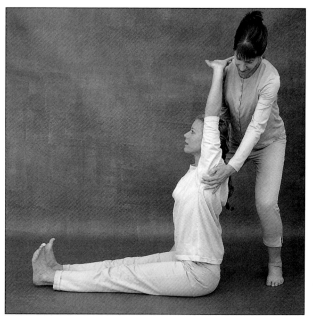
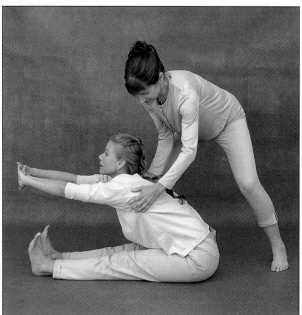
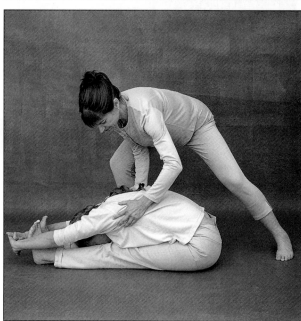

Gall Bladder and Liver Meridians

Your partner sits with legs wide apart and hands clasped, palms facing upward to prepare for the stretch. As she inhales, lift her slightly by holding her just below the arms and straightening your knees. This will lift her slightly out of her hips, but not off the floor. She will turn to face left, then stretch across her right leg, moving gradually on each of two or three exhalations. When she is in her maximum stretch position, lengthening toward the wall, not downward, step carefully in front of her left leg with your left leg and help her lengthen further to the side. You may use the inner part of your right leg against her spine to keep her sitting straight, rather than leaning rearward. This added support helps your partner gain the maximum benefit from this stretch. This is done only on her exhalation. Then, repeat this sequence on the other side. Remember, she will twist toward one leg, and stretch toward the other.

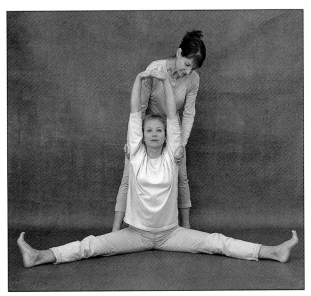
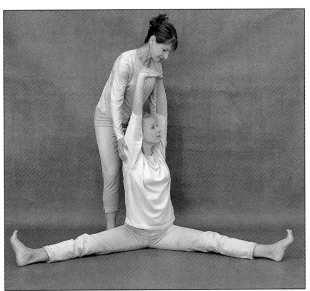
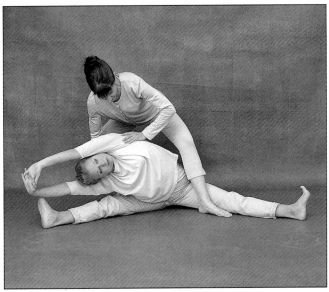

Small Intestine and Heart Meridians

Observe your partner as she begins to stretch forward. Your body is resting on the balls of your feet, one knee raised slightly off the floor. When your partner is in maximum forward stretch (after about three breaths), apply your knees slowly and gently on her back, just above the hips so as to avoid the kidney area, and your hands on her thighs midway between her knees and hips. With her next exhalation apply slight downward pressure on her legs as you lean slightly into your own knees. Release a bit as she inhales and re-establish pressure as she exhales, about three times. Release your contact before she sits upright again.

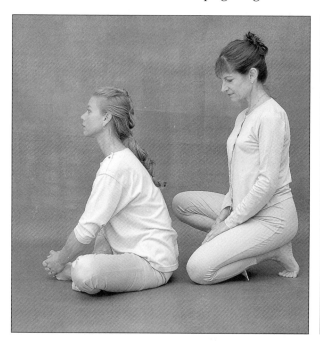
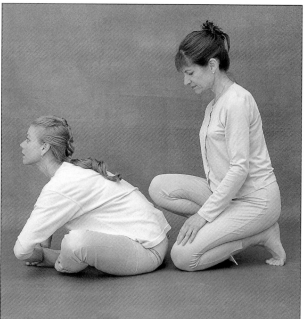
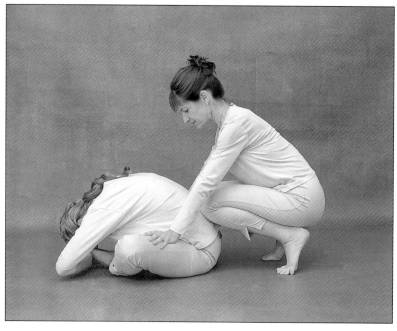

Heart Constrictor and Triple Heater Meridians

Your partner will sit with legs crossed and crossed arms, with her hands draped over her legs. Observe her body as she bends forward on the first exhalation. Drape your arms over her back and lean your body toward her. You may be on your toes to give you more mobility. She may stay in this position for three breaths, as you lean gently. Then, release your pressure as she sits up. She may reverse the position of her legs and arms and repeat the stretch, with you assisting again.

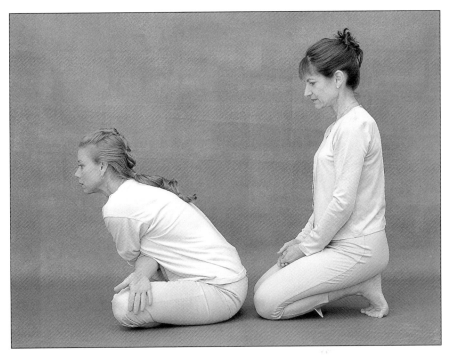

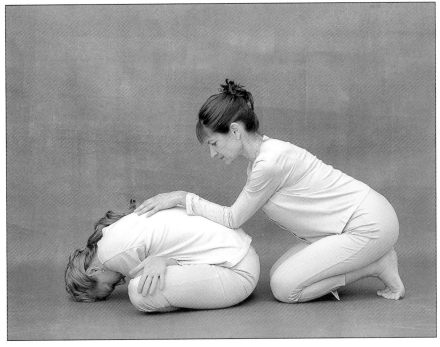

Stomach and Spleen Meridians

Hold your hands on your partner's knees as she begins to stretch back and downward toward the floor. You will notice that as she gets closer to the floor her knees may have the tendency to rise up, so keep a steady downward pressure. Each time she moves, it will be on the exhalation, however, do not release your pressure as she inhales as in the other stretches. Keep the pressure on her knees until she sits up again. She may then lean forward to stretch her back.

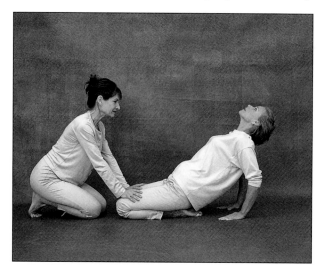

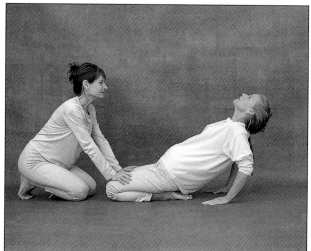

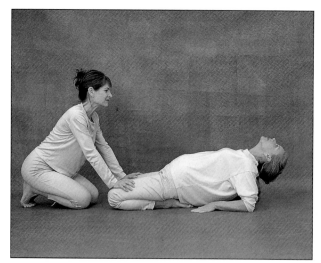

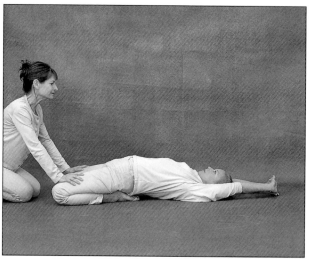

Extra fun stretch

Stand next to your partner, with the sides of your inner feet touching. Take hold of each other's hands, and with a wide stance, lean into your outer legs. Inner legs must be straight and the hands that are held overhead must be firmly clasped. Lean outward on the exhalation and support each other. Note that with this stretch you are inclined inwards but leaning outwards. Repeat on the other side.

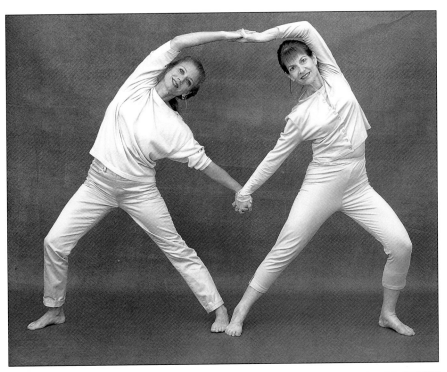

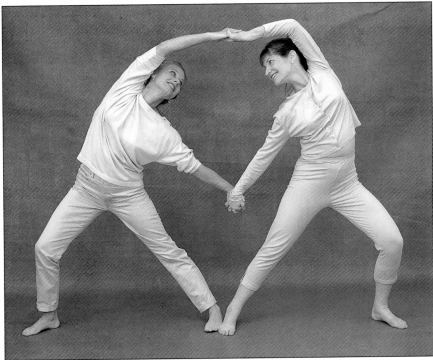

Preride Exercises for Riders

The following exercises will simultaneously stretch and strengthen your muscles, promoting physical balance. This is time well spent for both you and your horse. The brief beginning and ending movements will help keep you focused and centered. The entire sequence takes about ten minutes and will improve your riding and help prevent your horse from reflecting any side to side imbalance in your body. (I have worked on many horses whose riders were unknowingly causing their problems, and so have strongly suggested that the rider come to me for shiatsu for the sake of the horse. People who are often unwilling to look after themselves will do so if it is for their horse's benefit.)

You may wish to incorporate the preride sequence for your horse (*see* page 236); do this first, tack him up, and then do your exercises as he looks on. He will most likely watch you and listen to your deep rhythmic breathing, which will relax him further while he enjoys the work you have just done on him. This will surely promote a more harmonious ride for you both. After your ride, do the postride treatment for your horse (*see* page 236). Working on your horse will improve your concentration and flexibility. Do your preride exercises on one occasion *after* you ride, just to learn more about your body.

The exercises are performed standing, for safety and convenience, in the barn or outside. They may help you become more aware of your body and any lack of flexibility in some areas. Do them with inner awareness and patience with yourself. Even if you exercise regularly, do the movements slowly to avoid any sore muscles afterward. Pay attention to and respect your body. Remember that strength without flexibility or flexibility without strength can cause imbalance and set you up for injuries such as muscle spasms, pulled muscles, and other injuries that will take too long to heal.

If you wish to listen to me guide you through the preride exercises, and the preride and postride shiatsu techniques for your horse, you may wish to purchase my audio tape, *Shiatsu Exercises for Horse & Rider: Three Part Harmony.*

PRERIDE EXERCISES

Exercise 1 – centering

Stand with your feet comfortably apart and your hands relaxed at your sides. Breathe normally. Then deepen your breath slightly. As you inhale, bring your arms out and upward, palms facing upward, then overlap your hands overhead. As you breathe out, lower your hands slowly toward your center (just below your navel). Repeat this sequence about three times. You may also wish to visualize the gathering of energy and bringing it into your body. Keep your knees soft, not locked, your shoulders relaxed, even when your arms are overhead, and your breathing audible, so your horse may hear you and continue to relax.

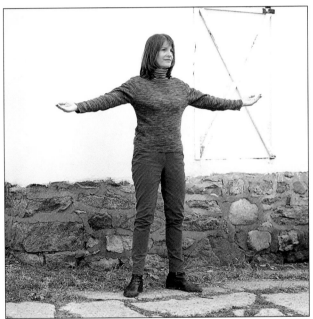
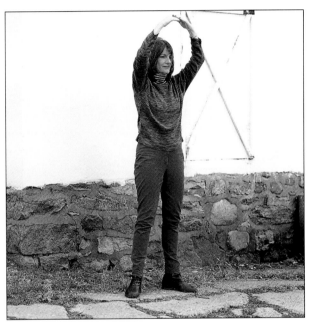
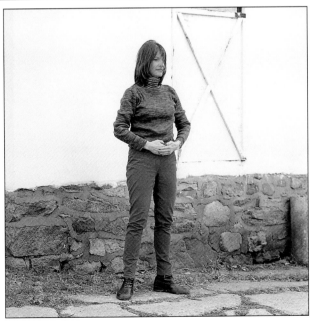

Exercise 2 – shoulder/arm rotations

This exercise is preparation for the following two strengthening exercises.

Pick up a grooming brush and hold it softly in one hand. Breathe in slowly as you take the brush forward and overhead in a smooth movement. Breathe out as you take the brush rearward and downward. This first circle should feel as if you are not using any muscles, rather, floating the arm from the joint. Repeat, this time stretching it forward so you feel the stretch in your back, stretch it upward so that you feel the stretch under your arm and through to the waist, rearward so you feel the stretch in your chest, and downward so you feel the stretch on top of your shoulder. Repeat, feeling the thorough stretch as you breathe deeply. Repeat on the other side.

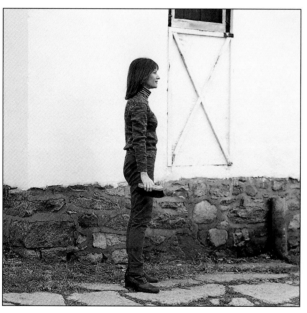
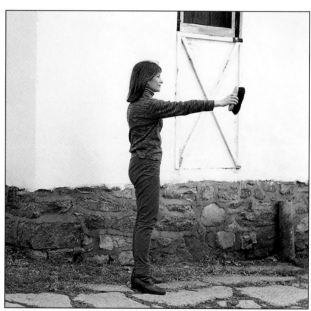
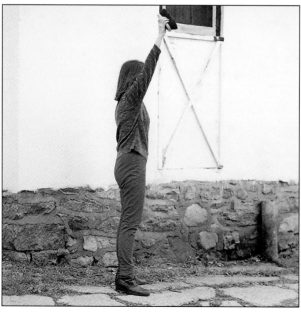
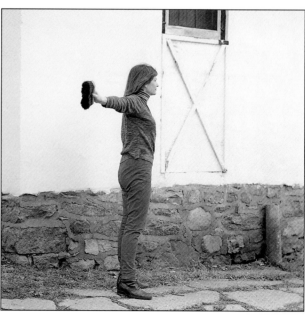

Exercise 3 – rope pull

This exercise strengthens the shoulders and improves posture.

Pick up a lead rope and hold it with your hands about shoulder width apart and with your arms resting on your legs. Breathe in as you lift it so it is in front of your chest. Breathe out as you pull on the rope for a few seconds (as if pulling the hands apart). Relax the tension and lower the rope. Repeat a few times, pulling on the exhalation. Pull hard enough so that you feel the muscles in your shoulders working.

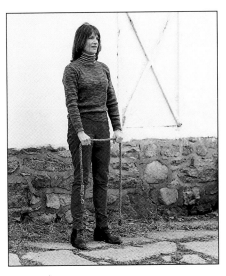 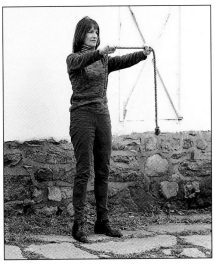

Exercise 4 – push backs

This exercise strengthens the chest.

Place your hands on the wall at about shoulder height and shoulder width apart. Stand about three feet from the wall with your body straight. Breathe in as you bend the elbows and go toward the wall, breathe out as you push away. Repeat about ten times. If you do not feel the muscles in your chest working, step a bit further away from the wall.

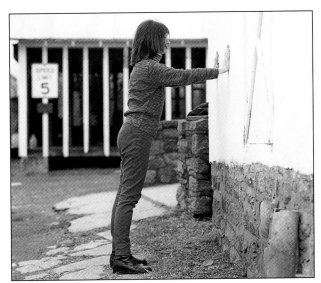 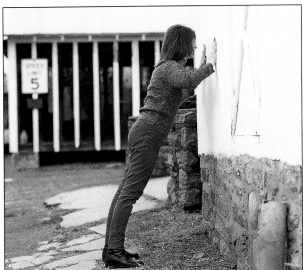

Exercise 5 – side stretches

This exercise strengthens and stretches the sides.

Stand with legs apart and arms out to the side *(top left)*. Tip to one side and hold your leg as the other arm reaches upward *(top right)*. Continue moving the arm so that it moves over and across your head, palm facing downward *(bottom left)*. Take the other hand off your leg, clasp the palms and stretch them sideways *(bottom center)*. Then, straighten up and bring the clasped hands overhead *(bottom right)*. Open the arms out to the side and repeat. Be sure to breathe with each movement. For example, tip sideways breathing in, breathe out as the clasped hands stretch to the side and reach upward. Repeat three times on each side.

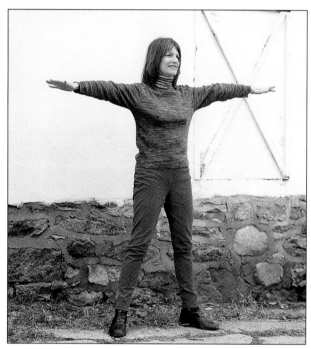
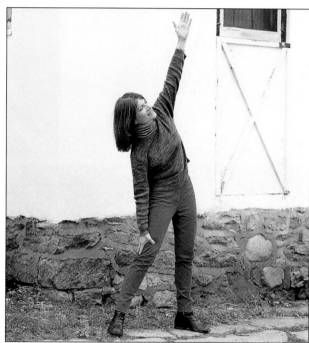

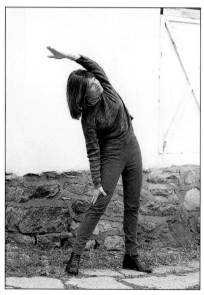
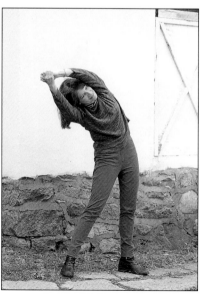
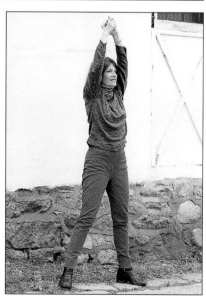

Exercise 6 – leg raises

This exercise stretches the legs, buttocks, and lower back.

Stand against the wall with your back as flat as possible against it. Lift your right leg, placing the right hand under and the left hand across the front of the knee *(top left)*. As you exhale, bring your knee as close as possible to your chest *(top right)*, then take it slightly toward the opposite hip *(bottom left)*. Inhale and release. Repeat on the other leg. Alternate from side to side, increasing the stretch a little each time.

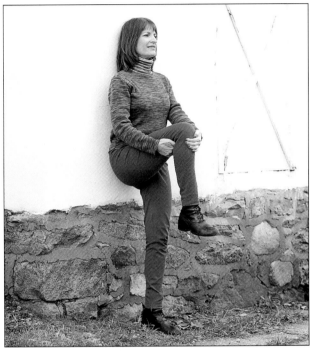

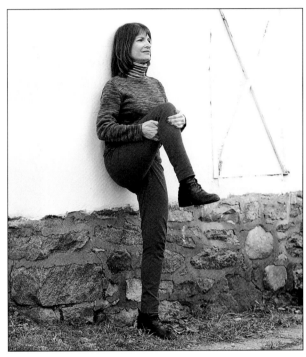

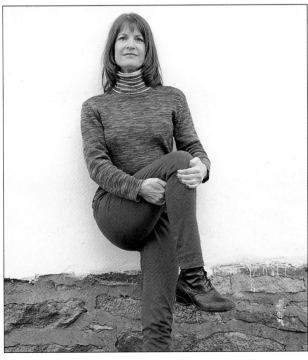

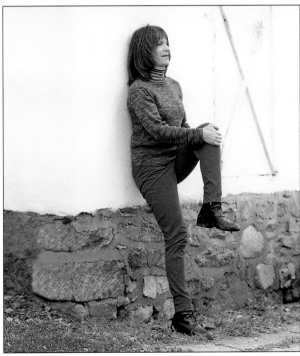

Exercise 7 – lunges

This exercise stretches and strengthens the thighs.

Take a long step forward. Drop your hips toward the floor. This will cause your rear knee to go toward the floor (do not let it touch the floor) and your front leg to bend at a ninety degree angle. Be sure not to let your forward knee extend beyond its foot. Straighten both legs and repeat on the other side. The downward movement should be accompanied by an inhalation, the upward movement with an exhalation. Repeat a few times on each leg, alternating sides. The more slowly you do this exercise, the more benefit you will receive.

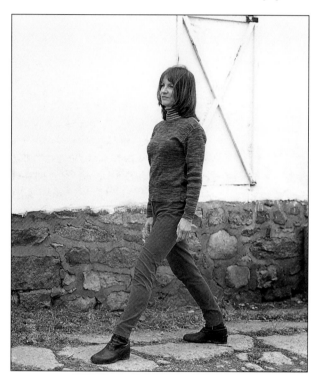 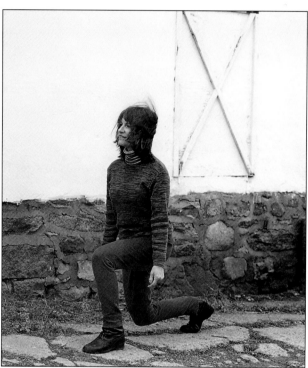

Repeat opening centering exercise for a few breaths.

Part II

EQUINE AWARENESS

Introduction

'Feeling' goes far beyond merely touching. Many practitioners can accomplish a lot from touching without feeling. 'Feeling' means that, when you touch an individual, you feel his or her life force. When you can do this, you can feel life. This is the most exciting part of shiatsu: touching life.

With this deepening of understanding, your touch becomes more meaningful and more effective; when you understand at this deep level, you become aware of a kinship among all living creatures. We are all expressions of love made manifest in individual form. With this realization comes a gentle, nonjudgmental acceptance of each other, in the present moment, and with the desire to gently help each other to realize our full potential. There can be no ego in this desire, only patient caring and gentle supporting action.

When you touch your horse, allow yourself to understand his life. Put your hands on him, let go of your thoughts and breathe with him. Follow the rhythm of his breath. Feel his life from within. Feel his life from his point of view. Try this with a few different horses, taking at least fifteen minutes to quietly breathe with each one. Let your expectations go and be in the present moment. You may be surprised by what you learn.

This skill may take some time to develop. Be patient with yourself, just listening to your own quiet breathing and letting your mind become still.

When you have practiced these skills, your shiatsu treatment can be like a moving meditation. You are following the life force of the horse you are touching/feeling as you are naturally led to each area that requires attention. You are reacting rather than acting.

This does not mean that your treatment is spaced out and ungrounded, or too airy. Moving meditation can be very dynamic or extremely quiet. Remember that you are responding to the needs of the horse you are treating, not your own needs.

When you work in this way, you will gain a deeper understanding of your horse, knowing better what it is like to be him. There is also an extra bonus you might not have thought of or expected: your horse will develop a better understanding of you.

Have fun.

Meditations

The herd

Sit comfortably, with your spine straight and, if sitting in a chair, with your feet flat on the floor and with your knees hip width apart. If sitting on the floor, sit cross-legged or *seiza*, that is, kneeling with your buttocks between your heels and your knees in front of you, about hip width apart. Breathe into your lower abdomen, letting it expand as you breathe in and relax as you exhale. Your chest does not move with the breath. Ignore any thoughts that come into your mind and concentrate only on the breath. Create a longer exhalation than inhalation. Continue to ignore any distractions, like noises, thoughts and body distractions and become the breath.

Imagine your present surroundings slipping away and being replaced by a large meadow. Smell the fragrant air and hear the peaceful sounds of birds, insects and wind gently blowing through the grasses and surrounding trees. Now you begin to smell horses and hear the sounds of tranquil grazing around you. You hear sounds of quiet communication and feel their telepathic contact with each other. You realize that your body as your body has ceased to exist and you are, in fact, one of the horses in this herd. You can smell the grasses as your sensitive lips seek out each bite. You know the exact location of each horse in your group without looking. You experience the feeling of dynamic relaxation as you placidly graze, always ready to take flight at the least signal of danger. Feel this interaction with your herd as you breathe.

After a few moments, or longer if you wish, let the scene and sensations go and begin to become aware of your surroundings and your breath. Notice how you are breathing. Notice your body and stretch a bit as you prepare to re-enter your own world.

Domestication

Sit in a relaxed position as described above and breathe into your belly. When awareness of your surroundings slips away, once again allow your imagination to roam free. Your body transforms gently into that of equus. You smell the smells of hay, water, other horses, urine and manure. Your surroundings are confined by wooden walls, ceiling and floor. You are aware of other horses around you but do not actually see them. Be willing to experience this situation. Presently a person comes in and leads you out, ties you up and goes through the ritual of grooming and tacking you up. Spend time experiencing each sensation in detail, especially bitting and saddling. Take your time with this. After the tacking up procedure, you may imagine the rider climbing into the saddle and riding you, then untacking and returning you to your stall. Pay attention to your breathing throughout this exercise, especially moments of tension, like buckling the girth, mounting and being ridden.

Initial Contact

GREETING

If you know that a horse is a calm horse, and your immediate surroundings are quiet, greet the horse by squatting in front of him and holding the lead rope. Let the weight of your relaxed hands draw his head downward, if he is not already intrigued by your humble posture. His head will lower, his ears will come forward and then you two may blow gently into each other's nostrils and begin to get acquainted. You may do this silently, or talk to him a bit. I usually ask the horse politely if he would like a shiatsu session (get him accustomed to the new word), then, ask him if I may touch him all over.

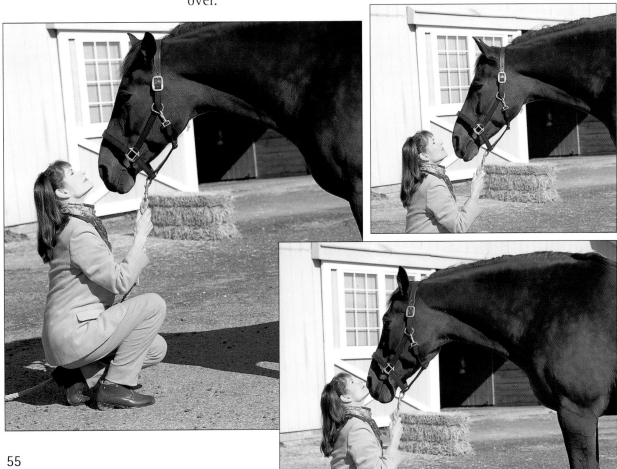

Chesa, a beautiful Thoroughbred, had been purchased by a woman who has since become my friend (I work on her, her husband, her dog and pony, and Chesa). Chesa had developed an injury in a front leg, which is why I was contacted.

Early on in the first session he made it clear that he did not want me to touch the leg, so I suggested that he be turned loose in the indoor arena. He ran around showing off for a while and I knelt in the center of the arena waiting patiently. In a few minutes he trotted over to me, stopped and gave me his hurt leg. We were then able to proceed with the work.

This magnificent horse, now twenty-one, is in fabulous condition owing to the excellent care and love he gets. He occasionally asks for me to work on him. He always teaches me something. In the winter he has the fuzziest white ears in the world. I feel he is one of the most communicative horses I work on and I listen carefully.

Now, stand up slowly and begin your first technique: stroking him all over his body.

ALL-OVER STROKING

Use your hands softly and smoothly, covering each portion of his body as your hands alternately sweep with long strokes. This is a medium-pressure technique. Begin a few inches down from his poll as the poll area may be sensitive, or a touch so close to his head may startle him. This is a calming introductory technique. Stroke down his neck, covering the entire surface, even underneath. Continue rhythmically moving your hands, covering his chest and shoulder and

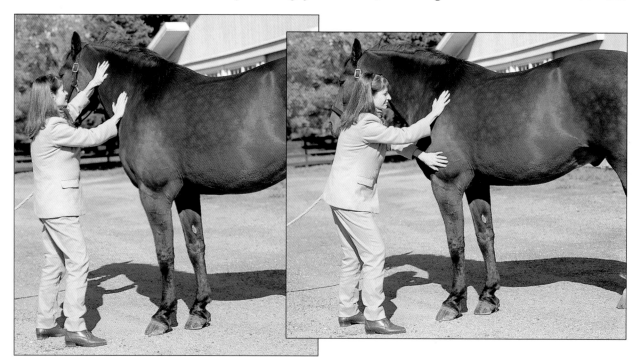

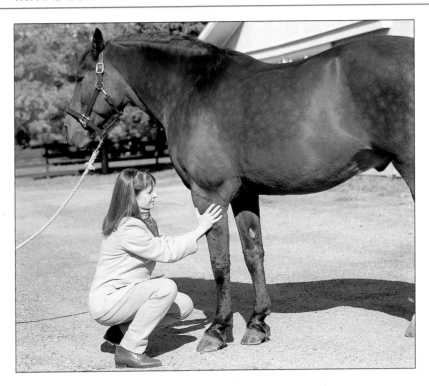

down his leg. Notice that I have bent my knees and lowered my body downward to finish the front leg. Work this way rather than bending from your waist and leaning over. Stand slowly and continue from the shoulder, across his back and barrel, toward his hindquarters and

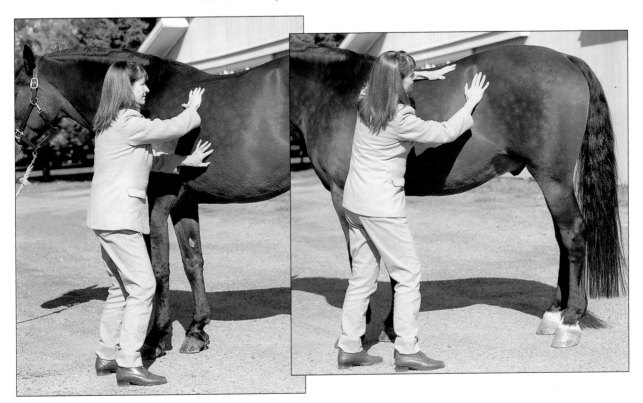

down his back leg. When stroking the legs, wrap your hands around the leg, covering the entire surface if possible, and smoothing down to the foot with both hands together. Finish by stroking the tail when ending the work on both of the horse's sides.

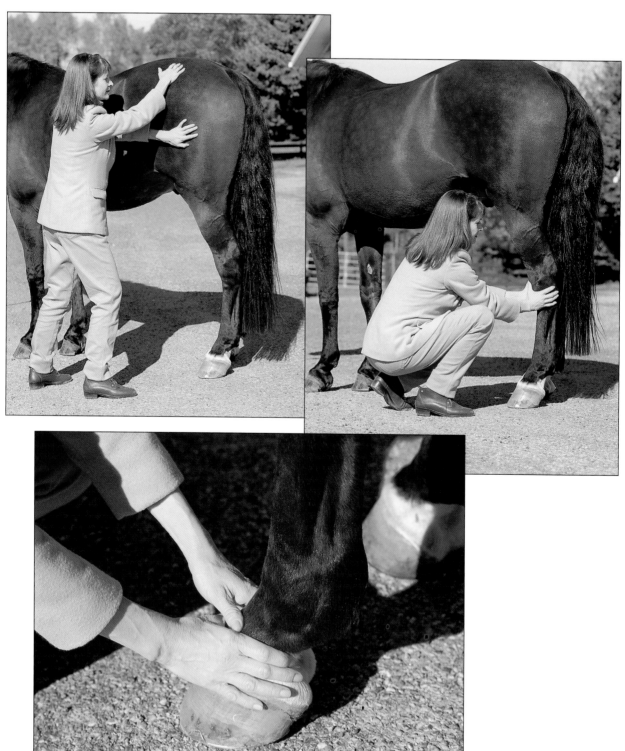

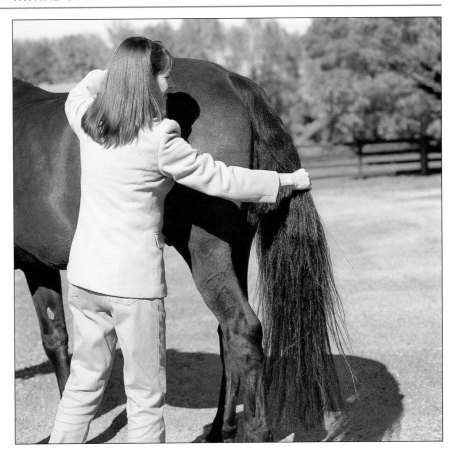

Notes and advice on all-over stroking

This is a technique that has many purposes. From the horse's viewpoint, it wakes up the nerve endings just under the skin. It gives him a sense of himself as a connected being, rather than a collection of body parts. It is also a very relaxing technique. If you begin and end each session in this way, your session will have a clear beginning, middle and end. Your horse will come to appreciate that this is the prelude to an extremely pleasurable experience. Use this technique even if you only have time for a brief session.

For you, this is a very valuable tool for obtaining information. First, you will sense the body temperature of the entire horse, with possible variations, which you must note mentally. Second, you will get a good feel for the condition of his coat, which is an important overall reflection of his general condition. Third, you will learn to quickly assess the condition of his muscles: toned, flaccid, stiff, tight, or perfect. This is particularly important as you stroke across the muscles next to his spine. If you feel anything less than balance, do not stop the movement of your hands, just keep stroking; we do not want to draw his attention to something that may hurt. You will make an overall assessment of his condition and be able to decide in what area to begin your first techniques (*see* page 60). For example, if you notice that his back muscles are stiff and tight, do not begin with back techniques. Perhaps work first on the hindquarters, or the neck, or do a few rear leg rotations, which will have a relaxing effect on the muscles of his back.

Amount of pressure

If you are working on a highly strung, temperamental or nervous horse you should match your energy to his at the beginning of the stroking. For example, this type of horse may become irritated if you begin a slow, soft stroking technique. I would use light to medium pressure and quicken the strokes a little, then perhaps repeat the procedure working more slowly as he begins to relax and respond. If working on a very calm, lethargic or sleepy horse who you may desire to wake up a bit so that he pays attention to you as you work, rather than dozing off and ignoring you, use a deeper pressure. Also, stroke more slowly in the beginning, gradually working a little faster as you finish the technique. In this way you begin by matching the energy of the horse at the start and then bringing his energy up or down in order that he may relax and physically and mentally participate in the session with you.

WHERE TO BEGIN THE TECHNIQUES

Following the opening stroking technique, you must decide on the area of his body on which to begin working. If he is sore or sensitive on one side of his body, always begin working on the other side. With a flighty horse, I begin working on his feet, doing rotations and point work on each foot starting with the front feet; this will help center and ground him. With a horse who is rather lethargic and needs waking up, I would do all the leg jiggling and rocking techniques, then work on the Bladder Meridian on the back. This will wake him up and help energize him a bit. Never do exactly the same routine on a horse more than a few times as both of you will become bored.

If working on an older, arthritic horse, avoid the manipulation (stretching, large rotations) techniques, as they may bring too much circulation to an already swollen and irritated area. Rather, do gentle and slow meridian work and perhaps a few jiggles to help loosen the joints. Proceed slowly and gradually, keeping your techniques simple and limited. After weekly sessions on this horse for a few months, he may be ready for some small rotations. After a few more sessions, if he seems comfortable and is showing positive results (less pain, more comfortable and fluid movement), perhaps incorporate a few small stretches. The older and arthritic horse must be brought along slowly and patiently.

If a horse is recovering from a leg injury, it may not be a good idea to do any leg work that requires him to stand on three legs. In such a case, do jiggling techniques and meridian work until he is comfortable supporting himself on three legs but, even then, do not leave him standing on the same three legs for more than a minute or so.

For horses with sensitive or sore necks, you will find that working on the hindquarters will likely release a lot of neck tension. If your horse refuses to let you touch his neck, as some of them do, try some neck jiggling. (This is sometimes accepted because jiggling does not involve pressure on the sides of the neck or controlled movement techniques. It is merely a loosening and freeing technique and most horses will accept a little of it. The crest is not usually painful so it is a safe place to touch; a horse may need to be held there for a moment prior to jiggling.) Then proceed to do five to ten foot rotations of the front feet, then try the neck again. If he still refuses to let you touch his neck, go back to a technique he likes better. Never finish the session with something you are unable to accomplish. If in future sessions he is still uncomfortable with neck work, you should certainly consult your vet. Some horses accept meridian work on their necks but not manipulation, so stay with the meridian work and do not ask for anything else for a while. The Triple Heater Meridian, throughout the entire meridian, is particularly good for neck problems.

Unsettled horses

For horses who have difficulty settling into a shiatsu session, you have to decide not only where to begin the physical work but also the best way to begin. You have many options.

The time of day is important; you may want to work on him after he has been ridden and he is a little tired. Make sure that the time allotted for the shiatsu session is well away from his regular feeding times. Remember that horses do appreciate their regular routine, so please try to fit your session in harmoniously.

You must also be very relaxed, so check your own energy level and make sure the horse is not unsettled because he is picking up on your level of stress.

It is preferable to work without a halter on the horse because this gives him the freedom to really express himself to you and show you where he wants to be touched, or not. Also, the halter does get in the way during the face work. If, however, you feel more comfortable with him in his halter, that is fine. You may even desire to tie him in his stall.

Should the horse continue to be restless, the next option is to work with someone holding him. The helper should not talk to him or touch him while you are working.

Tying the horse on both sides – cross-tying – is my least favourite option but it is a solution if you have a mouthy horse to work on and nobody is around to help you.

The ideal location for working on an unsettled or restless horse is in his stall, providing it is quiet and all the required techniques for the session can be accomplished in it.

Atmosphere, location and surroundings are of great importance to you and every horse you work with because you are equal partners in this endeavour.

CREATING AN ATMOSPHERE FOR HEALING

You want to create an atmosphere of peace and safety for you and the horse and the creation of a healing atmosphere first of all comes from within you.

Take a few minutes to center yourself before you touch your horse. You may stand near him or do this before you enter the barn. Stand quietly and bring your attention to your breathing. Begin to deepen your breath so that it begins in your lower abdomen. Relax your shoulders away from your neck. Your feet should be about hip width apart. This time is for the two of you so forget about what you must do after the session, or anything that happened before. This is a time of joy and sharing, so enjoy yourself.

Location and surroundings

Do not work on your horse in a noisy area where there is a lot of other activity such as horses being led in and out, stalls being cleaned etc. Let others who are working in the area know that you are working on your horse; they will hopefully keep the noise to a minimum. Turn off the radio unless your horse, like many others, needs music to help calm him. I recommend classical music. Just be careful not to get into the rhythm of the music, work to the rhythm of the energy of the horse you are with.

If you are working in your horse's stall, remove all the food so that it does not distract him, but leave the water. Only work inside his stall if the footing is even and you have enough room to do the stretches comfortably and safely.

CONTINUITY OF TECHNIQUES

Your techniques should flow smoothly, creating a beautiful flowing session, rather like a dance between you and your horse. For example, if you have just completed finger-pressure techniques along the front and rear borders of the shoulder and wish to do a leg rotation, bend your body slowly, keeping your hands on the horse, and lift the leg. Get yourself quietly into rotation position, and proceed. If you wish to do a foot rotation following a leg rotation, lower yourself downward smoothly and, without moving your hands around too much, place his foot across your bent knee. Always get your body in position first, so you can be ready to support the body of your horse. A session without continuity is choppy and distracting for both of you. Practice two or three techniques in a sequence to establish a graceful rhythm. For example, pick up the front leg and rotate, then, do a foot rotation, followed by the foot flop. Or rotate the foot, rotate the leg, and go into a stretch. If your techniques flow continuously you will both stay relaxed. You will not have to stop, break your concentration, and start again. Continuous movement will also help you to feel good after the treatment, as well as your horse!

Part III

SHIATSU TECHNIQUES

The Back and Hindquarters

BLADDER MERIDIAN

Bladder Meridian with palm pressure

Stand with your feet about hip width apart. Place one hand across your horse's withers: this hand we call the supporting hand. Place your other hand alongside it: this hand is your working hand. Both hands will be along the Bladder Meridian (*see* page 183), which you will soon be able to feel quite easily. The entire palm surface of your hand and the fingertips, will mold to the contours of his body, even though the only area exerting any pressure is the palm heel. Your fingers will be draped across the other side of his back. Be conscious of keeping your hands relaxed and not holding your thumb or any of your fingers up in the air. Lean your body toward your horse, dropping your weight into your palms. The supporting hand will press in gently first, followed immediately by the working hand. Hold both hands in the meridian for several seconds if your horse seems comfortable.

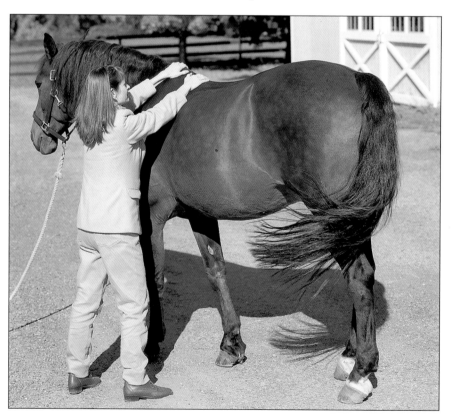

Notice that my right foot is slightly forward. This will be the case when your right hand is your working hand; when the left hand is the working hand, your left foot will be slightly forward. This position will create a good balance in your body, and you will be able to use the foot opposite to the working hand to push you toward the horse to create more pressure, if needed.

Next, release the pressure in your hands by shifting your weight a little rearward. Keep some pressure in your supporting hand (about half the weight). Move your working hand along the meridian about a palm's width from your first point of contact. Proceed in this way toward the croup. Lean your body toward your horse, sinking your weight first into your supporting hand, then your working hand. Hold the same pressure in both hands. On average, the amount of pressure applied to begin with, as you first begin to work, on a scale from one to ten, will be four or five. Work along his back until your hands begin to feel too far apart. Then move your supporting hand to another location, closer to your working hand, on the meridian. Proceed in this way until you reach the croup.

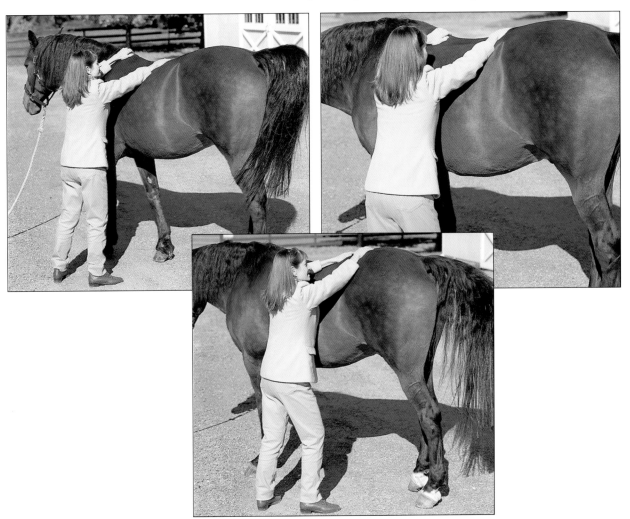

Take care that your pressure is not causing him to rock from side to side as you work the back. He should not have to constantly shift his weight to keep his balance as you work. You may have to adjust the angle of penetration to avoid this rocking. You should be pressing slightly more downward than across. If your horse is enjoying himself, repeat this sequence two or three times. It should take two or three seconds to sink into each location, and then hold for three to ten seconds, and take two or three seconds to release the pressure from each point. In other words, do not rush!

Fingertip pressure in the Bladder Meridian

Go back to your beginning position to start work with fingertip pressure. Your supporting palm will be across the withers as previously explained. Make a unit of the fingertips of your working hand. Round your hand and place the fingertips in the meridian. There is no space between the fingertips. Your palm may be lightly resting on his body if it does not tickle his skin. Work along his meridian with fingertip pressure, aided by your supporting palm, working slowly toward the croup. My entire body is relaxed, even my shoulders, although I must reach up to touch his back. My knees are soft, not locked, and my back straight. Try to maintain this posture, and smile!

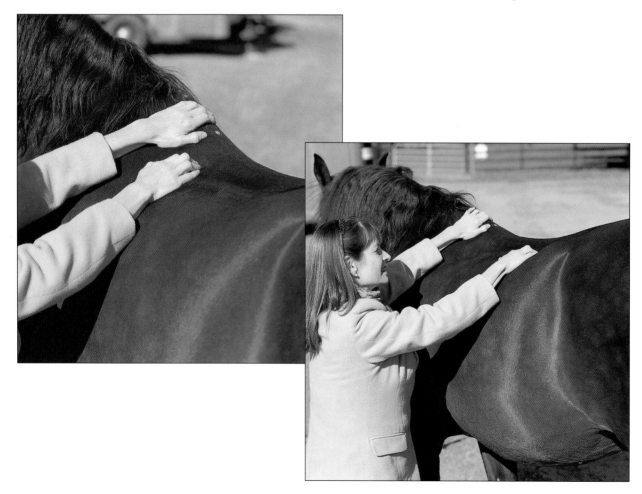

Bladder Meridian in the hindquarters and leg

When you reach the croup with fingertip pressure, continue from the croup to the dock with palm pressure and then with fingertip pressure. To continue along the meridian down the rear leg *(bottom right, and top left and right on page 68)*, change the position of your supporting hand, by turning it and pointing its fingers toward the tail. Your palm should be anchored just before the highest point of his quarters, this will keep it from sliding toward his tail. Also, change your body position so that you are facing toward his tail and step your foot nearest the horse rearward. Reach into the meridian with the fingertips of your working hand, and lean into your back foot. Simultaneously, you are pressing your supporting palm downward and slightly toward his tail without it sliding. The role of the supporting hand is especially important. It will keep him from rocking

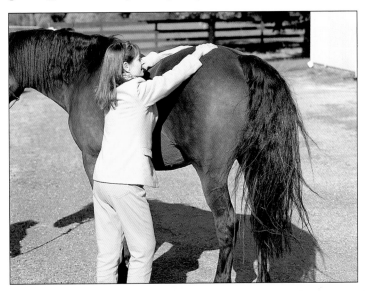

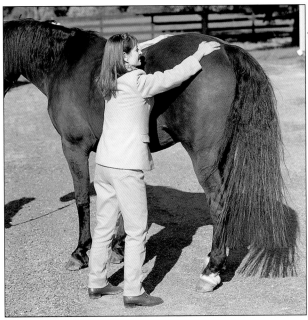

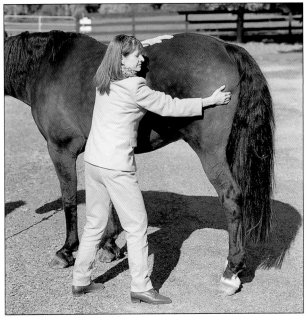

forward with each point you press along the back of his leg. Touch several locations down the back of his leg. Your hands will soon become too separated again as you get near the stifle, so slide your supporting hand down his quarters and his leg, and reach around the inside of his leg to place the fingertips of your supporting hand in the meridian; the fingertips of your working hand will be exactly below, in the meridian *(bottom left and right)*. You will create pressure by leaning rearward, into your hips, pressing in first with your supporting hand, then your working hand. Proceed this way all the way down the leg. If your hands become too far apart along the way, move the supporting hand again once or twice. Work all the way to the last point on the meridian, which is in his foot.

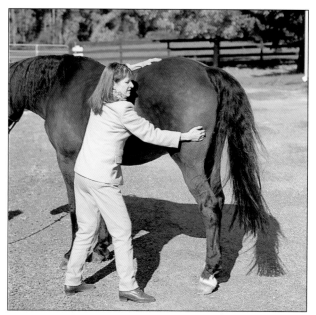
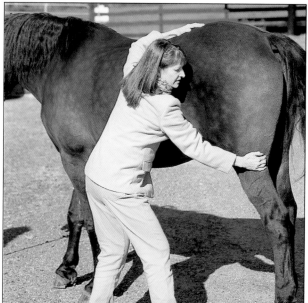
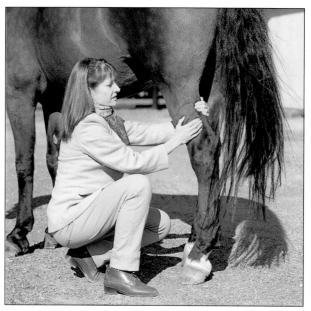
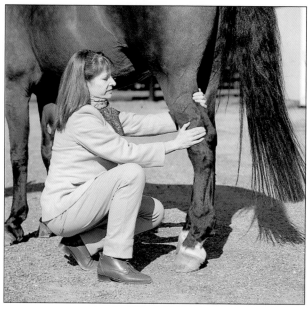

Working points in the hindquarters

Stand close to his body, facing toward his tail. According to your relative heights, reach up and across with your arm nearest the horse, by raising your arm up first, then placing your ribcage, then the entire surface of your arm, along and across his body. You may have to stand on your toes to accomplish this. The hand of this arm (which will be your supporting hand) is as far as possible down his hindquarters on the far side. This will support him as you work several points throughout his hindquarters. You should feel as if you are sandwiching his quarters between your hands. The supporting hand stays in one location as you work throughout the hindquarters with your working hand. Make sure he is not rocking from side to side as you work.

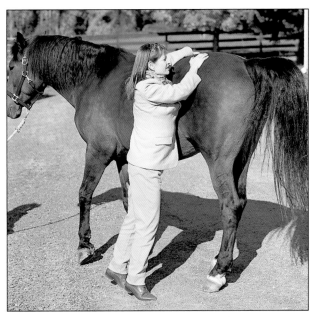
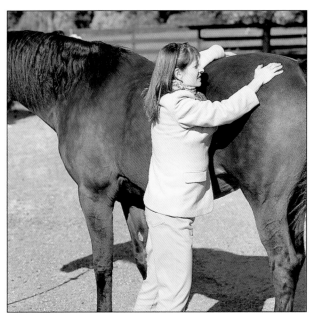
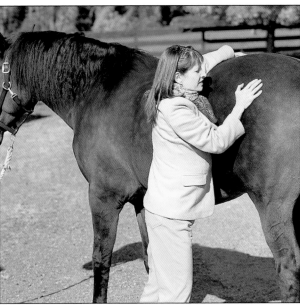
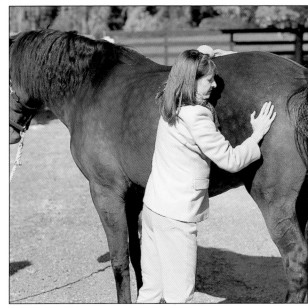

Bladder Meridian (second channel)

Place your supporting hand below the withers and your working hand alongside. Work the lower (second) channel (*see* page 183) of the meridian in the same way as the first channel following its location to the point where it joins the first channel.

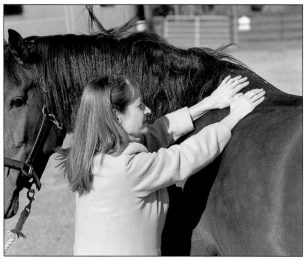
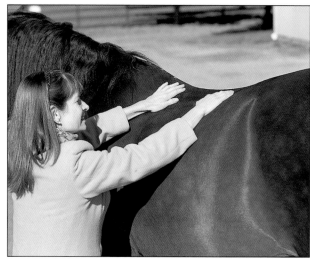

Bladder Meridian with elbows

For specific and solid deep pressure, you may wish to try working with the elbow of your working arm. Your supporting palm will take the same role as previously explained. Place the elbow of your working arm in the meridian with your arm nearly straight. Begin to bend your arm, simultaneously leaning toward your horse to create pressure; bending your arm enables your elbow to apply pressure into a specific point. The pressure, as always, is vertical to the surface you are touching. Hold for several seconds and then simultaneously straighten your arm as you shift your weight rearward to release the pressure. Work from the withers to the croup slowly with your elbow, moving your supporting hand once or twice along the way.

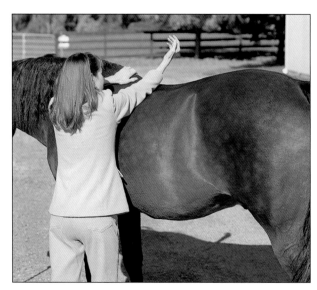
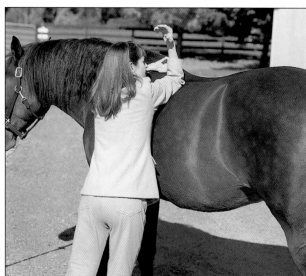

Bladder Meridian stretch Place your palms about twelve inches apart beginning near the withers (*see* right-hand photo on page 65). Lean toward your horse while simultaneously pressing downward with both hands. This is quite firm pressure, and should only be done after working on his back. As you lean in, push your hands toward his head and tail respectively, creating a stretch between your hands. Avoid sliding your hands away from each other. You will see the stretch between your hands. Slowly release. Take both hands along another twelve inches or so and repeat. You may do about three locations until you come to the croup. Stop there.

Alternative Bladder Meridian technique for the hind leg Stand behind your horse and take the tail in your right hand. Step back slightly with your right leg. Place your left palm in the Bladder Meridian. As you begin to lean into the meridian, offset the forward pressure by pulling the tail rearward. This way, the horse will not be feeling pushed forward. As you move along, release the tail pull as you release the pressure on each location of the meridian. Begin as shown and finish near the stifle. If you want more pressure, you may brace your elbow against your body and lean into the meridian with more of your body-weight.

Still using the tail to support the horse, position your hand so that your thumb contacts the meridian. Notice how the knuckle of my index finger is also in contact. This extra contact will offset the sharp feeling of your thumb. Lean into your thumb/knuckle as you pull the tail, creating balance. Hold each point several seconds. When using the thumb, it is particularly important to lean in very gradually, hold, and release gradually.

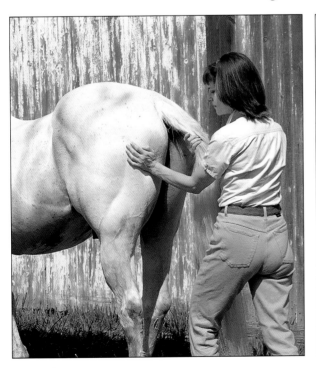
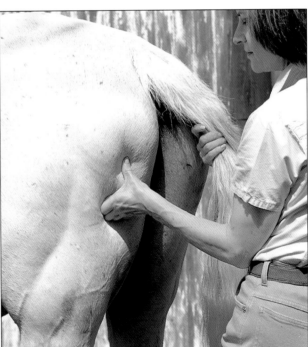

The Shoulders

**SHOULDER JIGGLE
(FRONT LEG JIGGLE)**

We always assess a situation before addressing it and the shoulder jiggle is not only a lovely assessment technique, it is valuable for loosening the shoulder muscles.

Squat alongside, but not directly in front of, your horse's front leg. Overlap your hands at the top of his leg just below his elbow. Bounce his leg lightly toward you and release several times without removing your hands from his body. Look at the shoulder muscles. You should see an undulating motion of the muscles as you bounce his leg lightly toward you. Start with just a slight movement until you begin to see some movement in the muscles, then, become a bit more enthusiastic to really get some motion. If he has a tendency to lift his leg when you pull, you may be pulling too hard so try pulling more lightly. If he persists in raising his leg, you may rest your knee on the front of his hoof, this will encourage him to keep his foot on the ground. Repeat this light, rather 'fluffy' motion from ten to twenty times in quick succession.

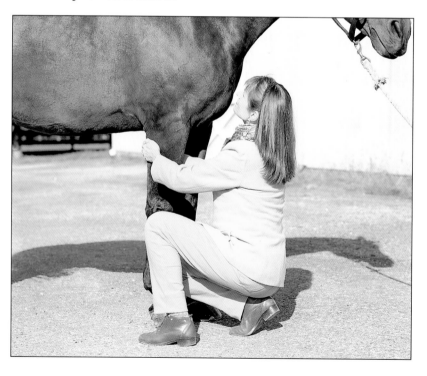

As you gaze at his shoulder, you must decide whether the muscles toward the front of his shoulder or toward the rear of his shoulder are looser. This will help you decide which area to work first. For example, if the muscles at the rear are looser (which they are quite likely to be), you will work on that area first as follows.

(Use this jiggle technique before and after the shoulder rotation [*see* page 86] as it will act as a monitor of the rotations' effect, or before any front leg manipulation technique.)

SHOULDER WORK

Place your supporting palm (in this case the right) across his withers slightly toward the front of the bone. Place the fingertips of your working hand in a space you will feel between the withers and the top of his shoulder bone. Work the next point along with the fingertips, tracing the outline of the bone downward for a few points. Then, using the side of your hand with your fingers pointing upward, press in and slightly forward toward his head. The supporting hand

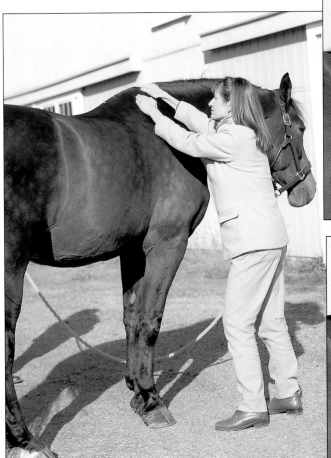

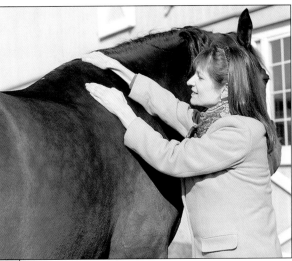

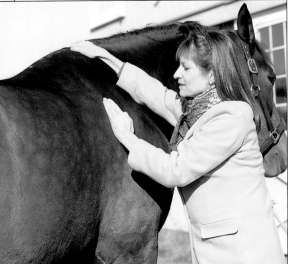

presses in first as usual, and releases about half the pressure as the working hand goes to the next position downward toward his elbow. Soon your wrist will feel overstretched, so change the position of your working hand; tuck your thumb out of the way against your palm *(top right)*. Then continue down his shoulder toward his elbow, really tucking your hand into his body if he is comfortable with this; your fingertips will be pointing slightly downward for these last few points and you will be using the index-finger side of your hand to press *(bottom left and right)*.

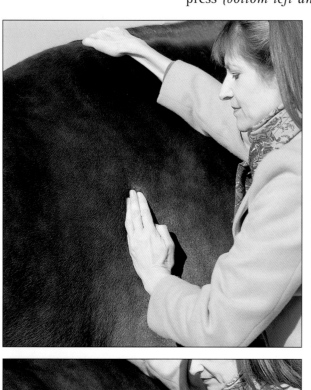

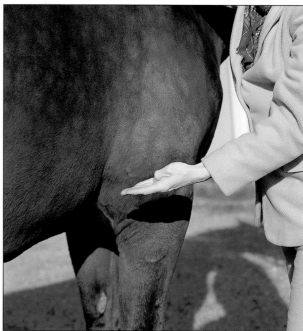

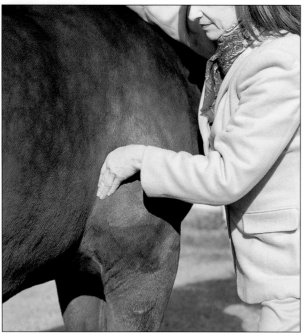

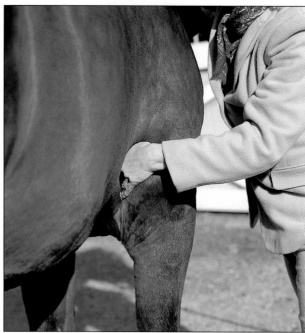

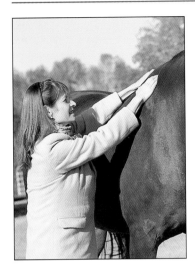

To work the front of his shoulder, place your supporting hand (in this case the left) across the top, and slightly to the rear, of the withers. Work the front portion of the withers with your fingertips as you did the rear portion of the withers. Continue down the area directly in front of his scapula using the little-finger side of your hand. Your fingertips are pointing upward and the surface of the hand you are using is the sides of the little, ring and middle fingers. In the next position or two you may feel a 'ditch' in front of the edge of the shoulder bone. You want to use your pressure to sink into this area, pressing gradually and gently toward the rear of the horse's body. When you are sinking in, bring your supporting hand down, with its fingertips pointing downward, and sink in with the sides of the little, ring and middle fingers of this hand as well. All your fingertips will be facing each other. Keep your supporting hand firmly in place

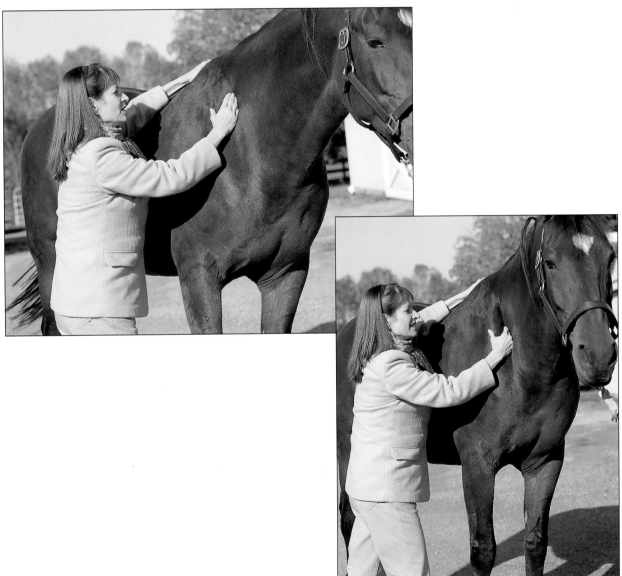

without releasing any of its pressure as your working hand continues down the front edge of the shoulder. If he objects to any points along the way immediately lighten your pressure. If your horse is sore in any of these areas, use very light pressure at first until he feels comfortable, then try to repeat the technique using slightly stronger pressure. Glance frequently at his face and ears for clues to how he feels about what you are doing.

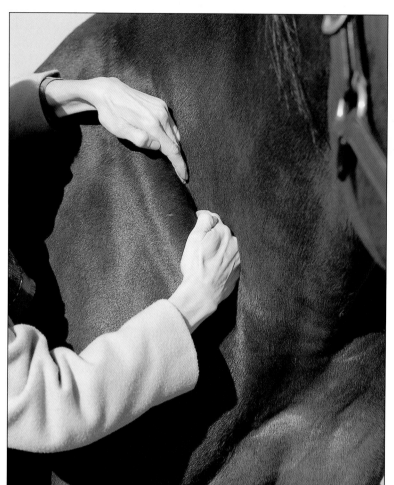
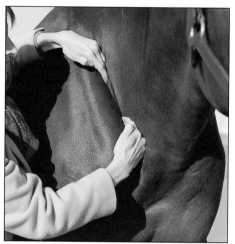
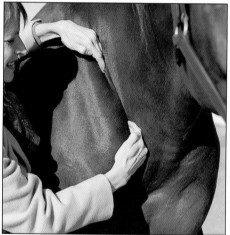

When working the rear position of the shoulder with your left hand, your left foot should be slightly forward. To achieve smooth pressure you should slightly twist your torso to the right. This will allow your hand to sink in without having to use your shoulder muscles and creating tension in your body. To release pressure from each point, untwist your body, place your hand in the next point and turn slightly again. To get your hand in the ditch in front of the shoulder, place the same foot as your working hand (in this case the right one) slightly forward, and twist to the left to achieve the desired pressure. Untwist to release the pressure, and repeat for each position. Working in this way your body will not tire, and you will avoid tension in your own shoulders. You will also feel more connected to the technique with your entire body. From the perspective of the horse, it feels much more secure and not painful as it might if you only used your muscle power. Always lean in from your center.

WORKING THE MUSCLES AND MERIDIAN POINTS OF THE SHOULDER

With your supporting hand across the withers, and using the palm heel of your working hand, work several points in the actual body of the shoulder, pressing gradually inward, holding several seconds in each location and slowly releasing. (If facing the shoulder, either hand can be the supporting hand. If facing toward the tail, the hand closest to the head will hold the withers. If you are more comfortable doing this technique facing slightly toward the horse's head, the hand closest to the tail can hold the withers.) If your right hand is your working hand your right foot is slightly forward, and vice versa. Mold your hand to the contours of his shoulder muscles. Your hand may actually feel as if it is filling up with the muscle.

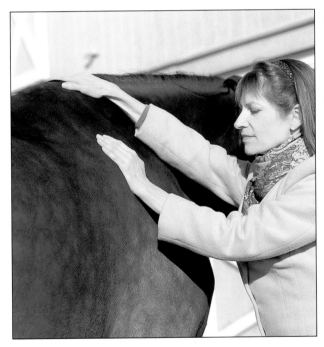
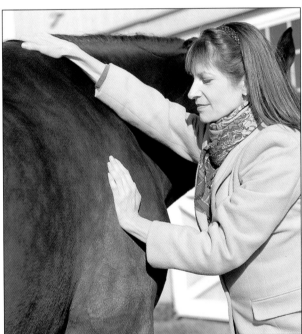

The Front Legs

MERIDIAN WORK

Use the following techniques as guidelines and adapt them to working on the Lung and Heart Meridians.

For a detailed reference to each of the following meridians, *see* Meridian Locations.

Small Intestine Meridian

Squat in front and slightly to the side of the front leg. Your upper hand is your supporting hand and your working hand is your lower hand. Position the supporting hand fingertips, which are close together, on the meridian by reaching around from the front and inside of the leg. Position your working hand just below it, from the outside, along the meridian. To achieve pressure, lean your body slightly rearward. Keep your back straight. Work along the meridian at regular intervals.

When your working hand is about halfway down the leg, move your supporting hand down to a point just above the knee, and continue toward the foot to the last point, just above the hoof, with your working hand.

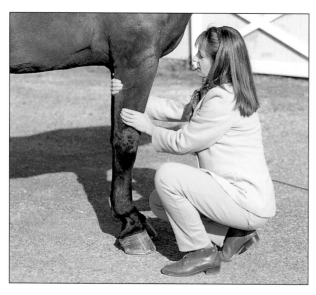
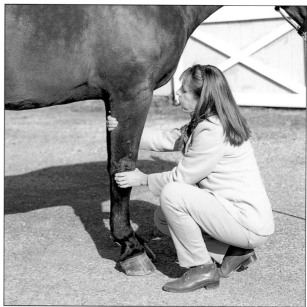

Heart Constrictor Meridian

Position your body alongside your horse's leg, facing toward the shoulder. Align your fingertips along the meridian. The upper hand is the supporting hand and the lower hand is the working hand. Lean back into your hips to create the pressure on the meridian. Keep your supporting hand where it is and continue down the meridian with your working hand. When your working hand reaches the knee area, place your supporting hand lower down on the leg, just above the knee, and continue working the meridian to the last point in the foot.

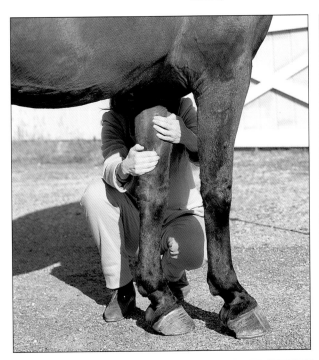

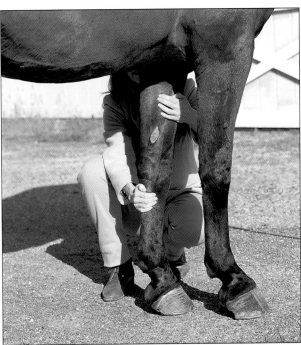

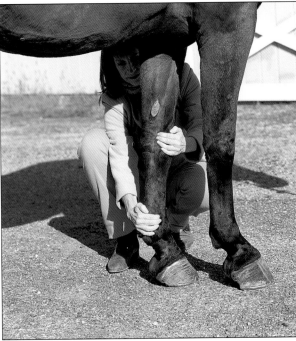

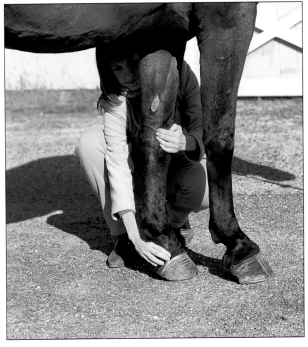

Triple Heater Meridian

Squat alongside your horse's leg, facing toward the shoulder (my position here has been slightly altered for the purpose of demonstration). Place the thumb of your supporting (upper) hand in the meridian at the top of the leg and the thumb of the working hand just below it. Proceed down the leg at regular intervals. *(Top left and right.)* Pressure is achieved by leaning your body toward his leg. When your working thumb reaches a point just below the knee, move your supporting hand downward, to a point just above the knee. Proceed in this way to the end point at the foot just above the hoof. *(Bottom left and right.)*

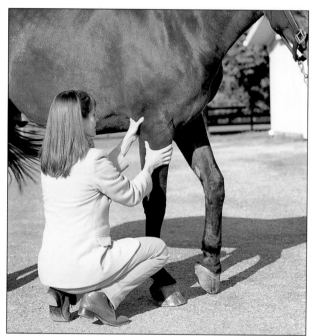
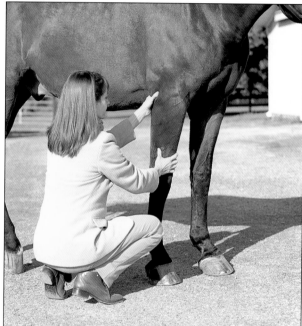
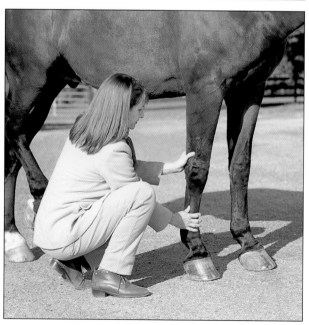
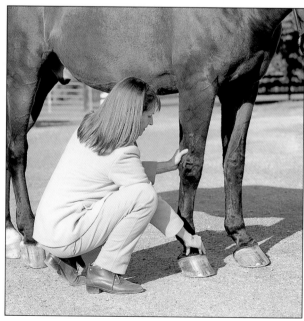

Large Intestine Meridian   Squat in front of and slightly to the side of the leg; your position will be at about a forty-five degree angle to the leg. Place the thumb of the supporting (upper) hand at the top of the leg in the meridian, and the thumb of the working hand just below it. Either hand may be the supporting hand but it will always be the hand closest to the shoulder. Lean your body toward the meridian to achieve the pressure. *(Top left and right.)* When the working hand reaches the knee area, lower your supporting hand to just above the knee. Continue working on the meridian, which is now wrapping itself around the leg to the inside, and proceed to the last point just above the hoof. *(Bottom left and right.)*

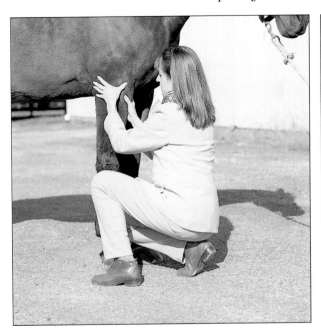
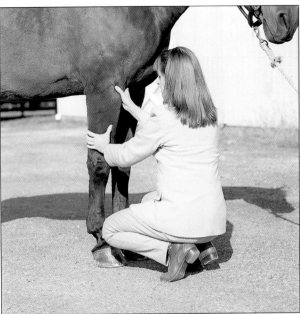
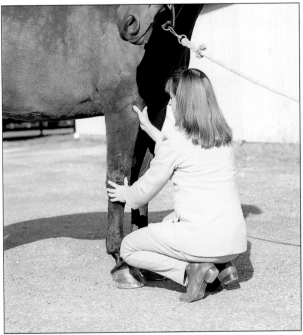
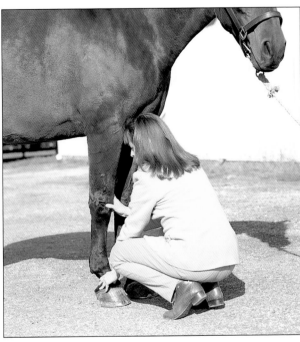

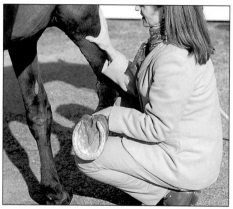 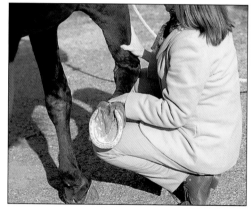

**Working the Small
Intestine Meridian with
the leg raised**

Holding the leg off the ground automatically releases tension in the
leg; hold the leg with the pastern across your knee, so that the con-
cave portion of his leg fits over your leg near your knee *(above)*. Your
knee should be inclined uphill so that he does not feel he will slip off.
Your supporting hand should hold him securely at the pastern. With
his leg positioned directly under his shoulder, not out to the side, work
from the top of his leg toward his knee with your thumb. You will
notice how much more deeply you can penetrate into the meridian
than when he is standing on this leg. For working the lower portion
of the leg *(below)*, use your fingertips to press downward, or the fingertips and palm to squeeze this area. Then, work some points around
the hoof before you replace his leg on the ground. To do this, hold
both sides of his hoof, stand up, then bend your knees with your body
alongside him, and place his foot on the ground softly (*see* page 84).

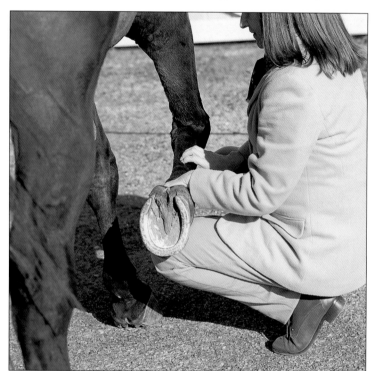

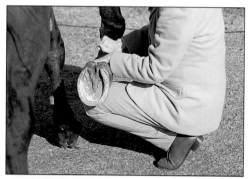

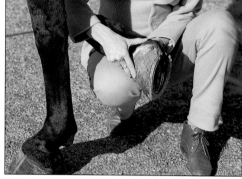

FRONT FEET

All these exercises will help support a normal range of motion in the foot. As with the shoulder rotation, you may also use the foot rotation for diagnosing the condition of the meridians. The techniques will also help your horse feel more grounded. In fact, on horses who are flighty and neither centered nor grounded, I may begin my session with foot work.

Foot rotation

Squat alongside your horse's leg. Let his foot (in this case the left) rest on your left knee. (Use either knee to support him according to what feels natural and safe.) He will be most comfortable if your leg is inclined uphill and the point of contact is just below his fetlock joint. Your supporting hand is extremely important and should hold his foot firmly and securely across the top, grasping with your thumb, fingertips, and palm, and also keeps his leg securely on yours; hold the toe of the hoof with the working hand *(left)*. Now, begin moving your body, to the side *(center left)*, rearward *(center right)*, to the other side *(bottom left)*, toward him *(bottom right)*, and to the side again while your hand rotates the foot. For the horse, this feels very different from that experienced if you only use your hand to rotate the foot. Your body should move quite a bit, even if his foot moves minimally. Notice if there is any restriction in any area of the rotation. Never force or strain, just support him. You may rotate in either direction, although you may find that one or the other feels more harmonious to him.

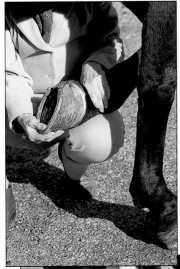

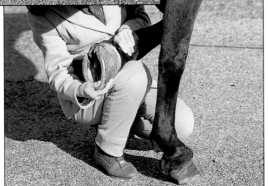

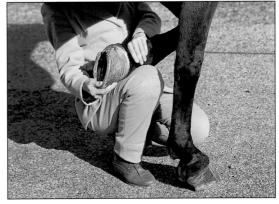

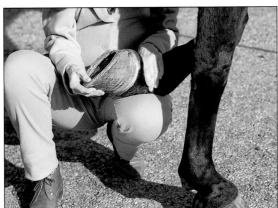

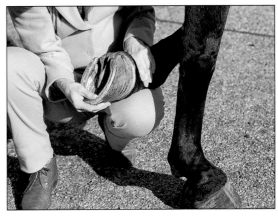

Lower leg stretch, to the front and rear

These two stretches should be done slowly, and *only* after the foot rotation. The second stretch (rear of the leg) may be difficult if your horse has a long leg, and if you have short arms, or if you are working on a pony. In such cases, just pressing the bulbs of the heel with your thumbs will accomplish the stretch.

Keeping his leg in the same position as for the foot rotation, as well as the position of your hands, lean your body toward his nose. This position will stretch the front of his leg up to his knee. *(Below left.)* Release the stretch slowly. Position your thumbs on the bulbs of his heel and your elbow behind his knee. This position will create a bit of traction between his knee and his foot. Lean toward the rear of the horse while pushing with your thumbs. This will have an effect from his foot to behind his knee. *(Below right.)* Slowly release. Hold each stretch position for several seconds. You may repeat these two movements two or three times.

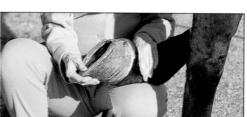
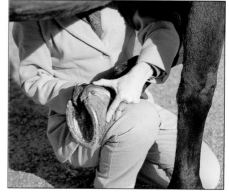

Replacing the foot on the ground

This technique is important because it keeps you in control of his body throughout every phase of the session. Rather than letting him snatch his foot away, or just letting it drop to the ground, replacing it in this way creates continuity in your treatment.

Move your inside hand toward the foot as your body begins to bend *(below left)*. Then, step forward with your outside leg as you move both hands to the foot *(below right)*. Finally, squat and take the foot with you, placing it on the ground.

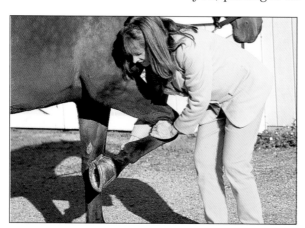
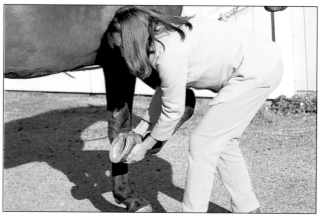

A treat for the feet

Most horses love this, as most people love a good foot massage. It is great for the circulation and you will be contacting end and beginning points of all six meridians of the front feet. Squat facing either toward the front or rear of the horse. Using all the fingers and both thumbs, work firmly around the coronary band and just above it, all around his foot. Your pressure should be quite firm and of medium speed. Watch him lower his head. This technique is a nice finale to the techniques of the shoulder and the front leg.

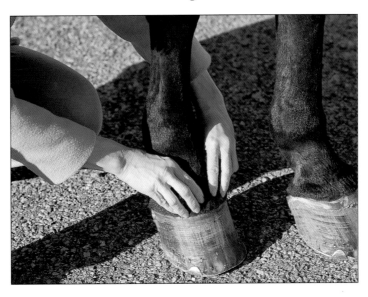

FRONT LEG MANIPULATION TECHNIQUES

For all of these movements, seek to establish continuity. Each technique should flow smoothly from the previous one. Only do two or three techniques on each leg before repeating on the other side. This will give the horse's supporting leg a rest. It will also enable you to determine the differences or similarities from leg to leg. Always go into the stretch position slowly and with great attention to the degree of elasticity of the muscles. By using your body to move the leg rather than forcing, you will be able to feel your horse's body more easily. Always hold the stretch position for several seconds, which will allow it to work to maximum benefit, and release the stretch slowly. Never force or strain, and keep in contact with your horse's feelings by listening to his breath and looking at his facial expressions whenever possible. The techniques stretch the leg bit by bit, in preparation for the full leg stretch. By stretching and moving the leg portion by portion, you understand exactly where your horse may be tight or resistant. In any of these movements, if you do feel tightness, work extremely gently and carefully. Remember, there is always another day if you are not satisfied with what you have accomplished. When you proceed to the full leg stretch, if there is any lack of elasticity, you will understand exactly what portion of the leg it is coming from. These techniques build on each other. You may change the order to suit the two of you, but always leave the full leg stretch until last.

Shoulder rotation

The shoulder rotation is versatile and will give you information about the flexibility of the shoulder muscles, the range of motion of the shoulder joint, and the meridian lines of the front leg. A small range of motion will help you to feel the condition of the joint. A larger rotation will help you understand the condition of the muscles. As you rotate, moving your body from your center and taking the leg with you, be thinking of the location of each meridian. Note that during the forward part of the rotation, the meridians at the rear of the leg are being slightly stretched (Heart and Small Intestine). As you rotate the leg away from his body, you are feeling the meridian on the inside of his leg (Heart Constrictor). As you rotate his leg rearward you are feeling the meridians in front of the leg (Lung and Large Intestine), and as you take his leg inward toward his other leg you are feeling the meridian on the outside of his leg (Triple Heater).

Cradle his leg (in this case the left) in your hands. Your left arm

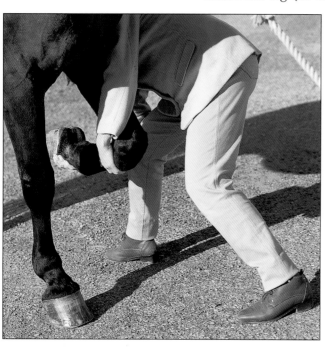

reaches around from the front of his leg to hold him under his knee. From the outside of his leg, your right hand supports the pastern. His lower leg should be parallel to the ground. You are facing toward his shoulder from the front of the horse. Take a wide stance. Moving from your center, lean into your right foot, taking his leg with you, then lean forward moving his leg backward toward his tail. Lean into your left leg, moving his leg a little toward his other front leg, then lean rearward taking his leg forward toward his nose.

You will be taking the leg along on a smooth rotation. Move slowly, giving him the full benefit of the movement. You may rotate in either or both directions. You may notice that one direction or the other feels more harmonious to his body. In this case, rotate only in this direction.

Upper leg diagonal stretch

This stretch is particularly good for dressage horses as it will help stretch the muscles used in crossover techniques and any free-flowing movements of the front legs.

Pick up the leg and then squat facing toward the shoulder. For working the right front as shown here, cradle the leg in your left hand, holding the foot. Your arm is resting along your thigh, and your wrist is off your knee. Your right hand is in front of the leg just above his knee. Then, using the palm of your right hand as the contact point, lean your body toward him, to create a diagonal stretch of the upper outside portion of the leg *(opposite, top left)*. Without letting go, bring the leg into a neutral position by moving your body into its beginning position. Then, using the fingertips of your right hand as the contact on the inside of his front leg, lean your body rearward, creating a diagonal stretch of the inside of his front leg *(below right)*. Hold each of these positions for five to ten seconds to allow him to connect with the movement physically and mentally. In either of these positions, the hand holding the foot is just a support, it does not move. Still holding the leg, now back to its neutral position directly under his shoulder, grasp him above the knee with your right hand, thumb on the outside, fingertips on the inside. Then, using a rhythmically flowing motion, which will be initiated from your body, not just your hand, loosely swing his knee toward and away from you, creating a relaxing effect on the shoulder muscles. Look at the shoulder to see the movement of the muscles.

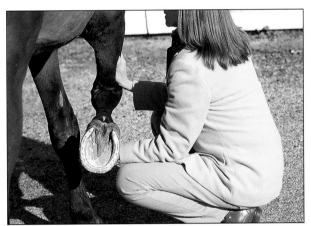
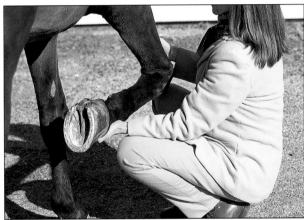

Upper leg stretch for Heart Constrictor and Triple Heater Meridians

This movement is beneficial for dressage horses.

Cradle the leg in both hands. One hand is under the hoof or pastern, the other under the knee. Stretch the inside of the leg by leaning rearward and taking the leg with you *(below left)*. In this case, both hands are pulling equally. To stretch the outside, lean your body toward him *(below right)*. The push comes through both hands equally. Hold each of these positions several seconds, and always release slowly. You may return his leg to the ground or proceed to the next technique.

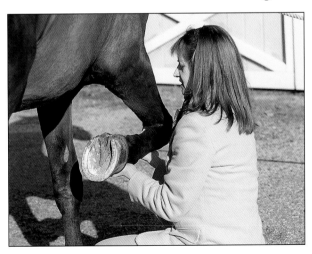
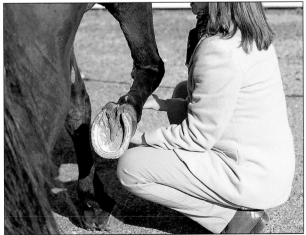

Knee exercise

This technique is good for all horses but be especially careful with older horses as they may have very stiff knees and be arthritic. Go slowly and only seek to reinforce the existing range of motion rather than increase the movement too much in the older stiff horse.

Cradle the leg in both hands as shown. Slowly raise the lower leg. Do not let the fetlock joint bend, keep the lower leg straight. You are bringing his foot toward his elbow, not lifting his knee. Hold the leg still at the first point of resistance, then release slightly, and raise it again. Release and raise the leg a few more times. Be aware of the degree of elasticity or tightness, and never force the stretch. This movement also stretches the upper portion of the Large Intestine Meridian.

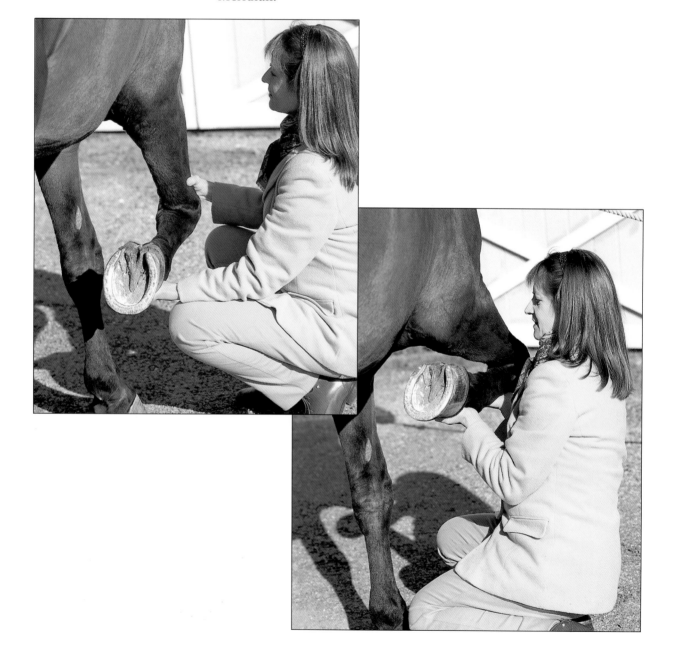

Foot flop

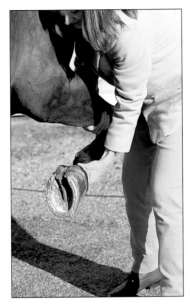

This is a wonderful release technique. It may be done after you do the foot rotation (*see* page 83). It is good for releasing tension in the fetlock joint of any horse. It gives the horse an unusual sense of his body as his foot loosely flops while you support his leg. Pick up the leg, in this case the right front, and place your right hand under his knee from the inside, hold his foot firmly with your left hand *(left)*. Working quickly but not abruptly, place his lower leg on your right thigh *(bottom left)*. His fetlock joint should be resting in the soft spot just above your knee. Your thigh is bent to support the weight of his leg. As soon as he is comfortable resting his leg on yours, remove your left hand from his foot and overlap the right hand with it *(bottom right)*. You are now supporting his leg with both hands and your bent leg. If he feels secure (you will feel the contact of his entire lower leg resting on your thigh), slowly straighten your supporting leg, letting his hoof point toward the ground. Begin to rhythmically bounce your leg, keeping your heel on the ground. Your knee will be going forward and back. This should set up a motion in his foot that lets it flop freely if he is relaxed. It is a free and bouncy technique. It may take you a bit of practice to get the rhythm just right and for your horse to let all the tension out of his foot. The technique is a good monitor of how successful you are with the foot rotations.

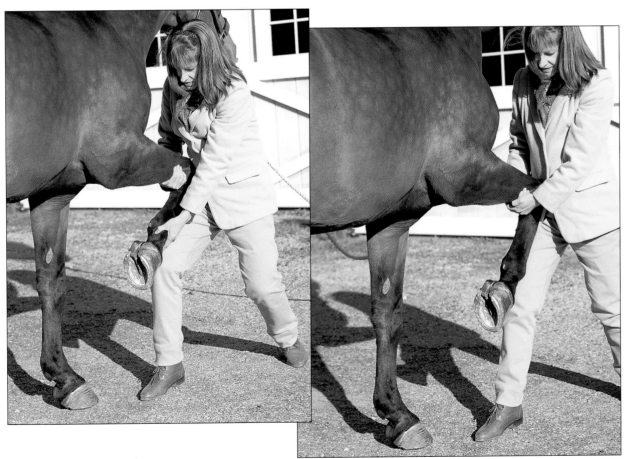

Shoulder release

This technique follows on nicely from the foot flop. It is good for releasing tension in the rear portion of the shoulder and will help your horse lengthen his stride. It is also very good preparation for the full leg stretch.

After the foot flop, remove your left hand from behind the knee and place it on his lower leg. Use your hand to push his leg between your thighs; close your knees so that his foot is firmly and securely held between your thighs *(left)*. Then, bend your knees; supporting him firmly with your right hand behind his knee, place your left hand behind his shoulder muscle, press in gently but firmly with your fingertips *(center left)*. Straighten your knees and you will feel this area stretch slightly *(center right)*. Then, place your fingertips a bit lower down the shoulder as you bend your knees again *(bottom left)*. Press in firmly with your fingertips and straighten your knees *(bottom right)*. This gentle stretch and release movement may be repeated several times as your working hand (in this case the left) works its way down the rear portion of the shoulder.

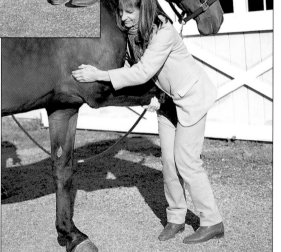

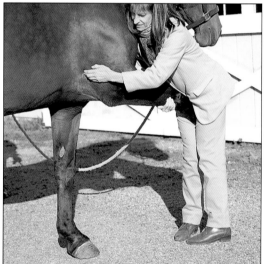

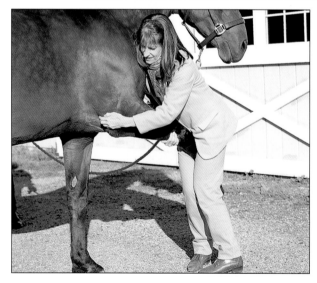

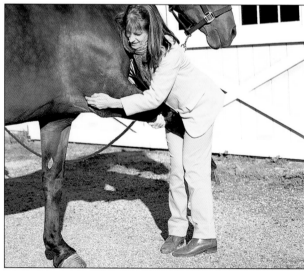

Shoulder rocking

This is a great technique for releasing tension in the deep muscles of the shoulder. His leg is completely supported by you and you will be stretching and releasing the muscles of the shoulder and upper leg both front and back. It may even help your horse if he has sore withers. The technique is good for any horse, however, jumpers in particular will benefit from it. Please note that this technique works according to the relative sizes of you and your horse. A very small person working on a very tall horse may not be able to accomplish this technique.

Hold his right front leg with your left hand under his pastern, the other hand at his knee. Bend your knees to lower your body and place his knee at the top of your thigh where it meets your hip *(left)*. There is a nice indentation here where his knee will fit comfortably. Use your right hand to keep him secure in this position. Then, straighten your legs as you simultaneously raise your right hip upward, taking his knee with you *(right)*. This hip movement is a sort of dance movement and works best if you have flexible hips. Hold his leg in this position for several seconds. Then, pivot on your feet to face the rear of the horse

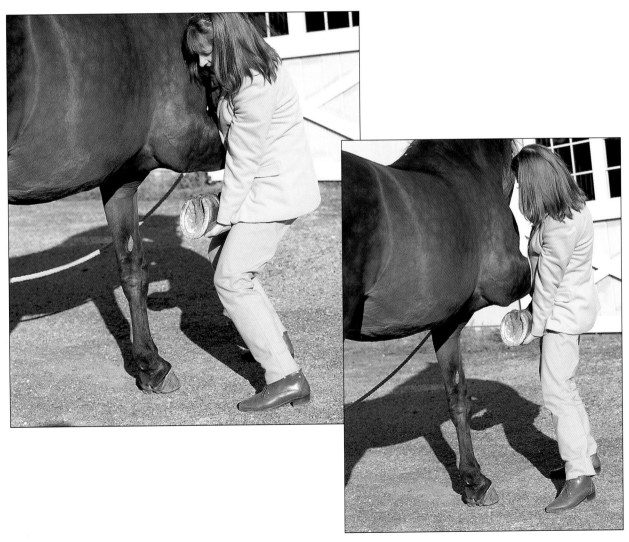

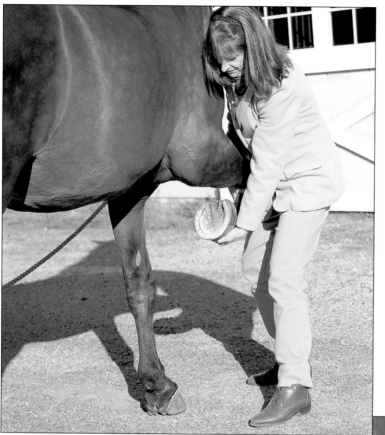

as you allow his knee to slide from the crook in your hip and leg, along the front of your thigh *(left)*. When his knee is about halfway down the front of your thigh, lean your body forward (toward the rear of the horse), thereby stretching the front of the upper leg, and compressing the area behind his shoulder that you just stretched *(bottom, left and right)*. Repeat this sequence several times: turning to face his shoulder, placing his knee in the crook of your hip, swinging your right hip upward and taking his leg with you, pivoting, and letting his knee slide securely to your front mid-thigh, and leaning into your left foot. Replace his foot on the floor by placing one hand on each side of his hoof and bending your knees.

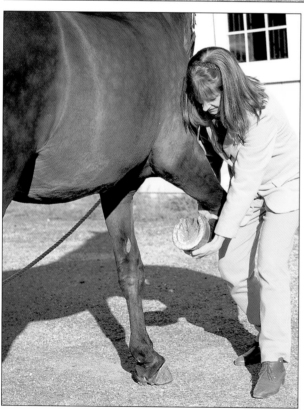

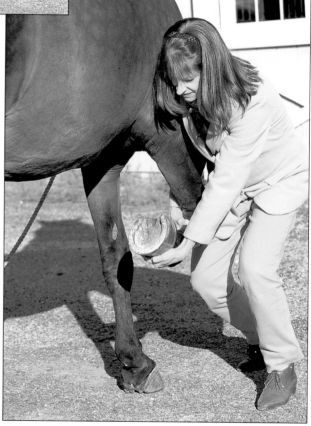

Full leg stretch

This stretches the muscles behind his entire leg, shoulder and withers. It should be done only after preparation with several of the above techniques. All horses will benefit from this, especially horses who are asked to lengthen their strides.

You may decide to move from the previous technique directly into this one. If so, do not replace his foot on the ground but keep holding the leg off the ground. Position your left hand behind his knee from the outside and step rearward with your right foot. Place your right hand beneath his fetlock joint. His leg will straighten. Do not pull his leg. Rather, hold him in this position for a few seconds, then lean your body slightly rearward. Stop leaning before you feel tension in his leg. Hold this position. If he feels good and confident and wants to stretch more, he will lean rearward. In the rare event that your horse begins to lean toward you, immediately shift your weight into your front foot, remove your hand from his foot and push the front of his shoulder to let him know he should lean rearward. Here *(left)* I am standing to stretch his leg. This position will stretch the rear of his shoulder and the back of his leg. Here *(right)* I am squatting and leaning rearward. This stretch will affect him all the way up to the withers. To release the stretch, shift your weight into your left foot, bend his leg using the hand that is supporting his foot, place one hand on each side of his hoof, bend your knees, and replace his foot on the ground.

Do not let him snatch his leg from you. To avoid this, learn the technique well by studying the choreography without actually trying to stretch him. You should try to sensitize yourself to his energy so you stop leaning just before he decides that he has had enough. You always want to have his confidence. If he becomes insecure and unbalanced during any of these movements, it may take some time to re-establish his trust in you. Therefore, go slowly and always remember that tomorrow is another day.

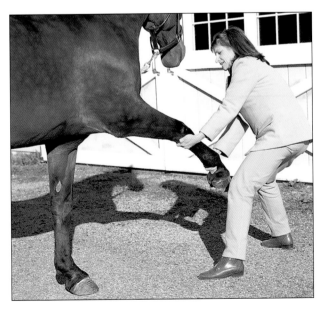
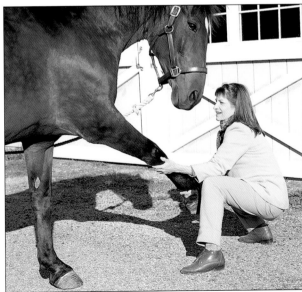

Variations of the full leg stretch

You may adjust the full leg stretch to stretch specific meridians. For example, from stretching the leg directly in front of his shoulder as explained in the previous technique, take his leg gradually across toward his other shoulder *(top)*. This will stretch the Small Intestine Meridian. Taking the leg from its forward stretch position and stretching it slightly away from the other leg will stretch the Heart Meridian *(bottom)*. Please take careful note of my body position in each photo. You must position yourself each time so that all you have to do to create either of these stretches is to lean your body gradually rearward. As always, slowly release the stretch and quietly return his foot to the ground.

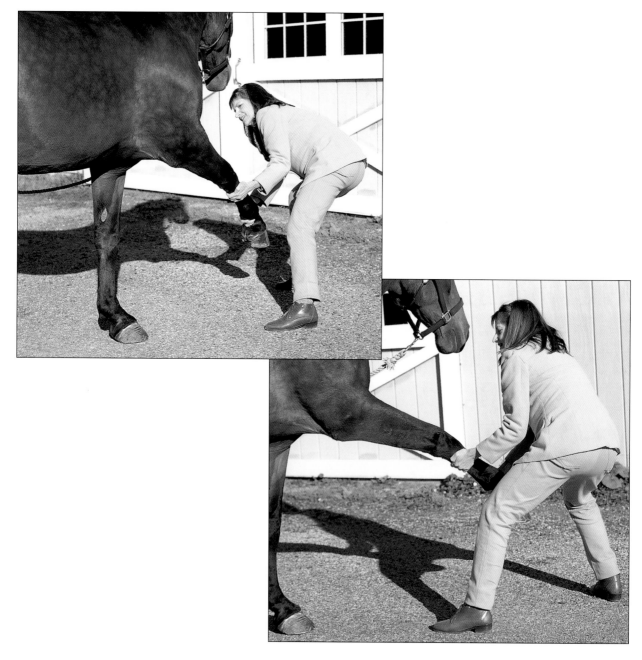

The Back Legs

BACK LEG JIGGLES

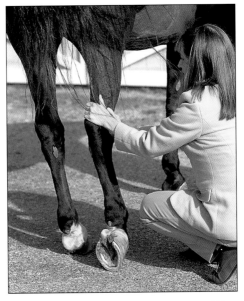

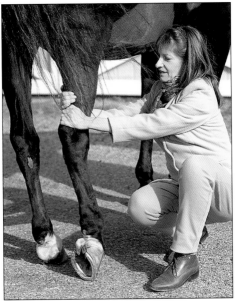

These two movements should be done before any manipulation of the back leg (as with the shoulder/front leg jiggle) since they are very good preparation techniques for rotations and stretches. These two loosening techniques are beneficial for any type of horse but especially those with tight muscles in their hindquarters. They are wonderful release techniques and you will see the muscles in the quarters loosening and undulating in the well-muscled but flexible horse. You may notice very little movement at all in the horse with stiff muscles. You may also feel restriction of the joints of the rear leg if the movement seems jerky. It is very important to use your body to create what is a loose rocking motion, a swinging motion. You may have noticed that the muscles in the hindquarters were very tight when you were working on the Bladder Meridian and various points in that area. In that case, you may expect a slightly restricted movement during the jiggle. However, if you did a very good job working on points in the quarters, the muscles may be moving freely now. As with all other techniques, this will help you assess the condition of this area of his body.

Encourage your horse to rest on his toe. Squat facing the side of his leg. Place one hand on the top portion of the hock on the rear of the leg and the other hand across the front of the leg, and in front of the other hand. Moving from your center and using your body and the hand that is on the hock, rock his leg to and fro rhythmically, creating a swinging motion that carries up through all the muscles of his quarters. Keep rocking, becoming more or less enthusiastic according to his response. His toe should stay where it is on the ground.

Then, pivot on your toes to face toward his tail. The hand that is on the hock does not move. The other hand reaches around from the inside of his leg and holds the leg just above the hand that is on the hock. Begin to bounce his leg lightly toward you, letting it release back each time naturally. Continue this rhythmic motion, from your center, several times, and you will feel the loosening and releasing of the muscles of the rear of his hindquarters, and especially the hamstrings.

If your horse is reluctant to rest on his toe, consider that he may not be comfortable supporting himself on the other leg. Work on the sensitive supporting leg first then try the other leg again. If he still will not rest the leg on its toe and you suspect sensitivity in the quarters or leg on the other side, work a little on the meridians and try to find the painful places by feel and gauging his reactions on the suspected sensitive side. If, after this, he will still not rest one or both legs, leave the techniques that involve resting on the toe, or any techniques that involve supporting himself on one back leg, until another day.

BACK FEET

Leg lift and foot rotation

This method of lifting the leg is much easier than trying to pick it straight up with just your hand. The foot rotation is good for all horses, however I particularly like it for jumpers; so many of them knock jumps with their back feet that I wonder if they have a sense of their feet at all. The stretches that follow this technique will also enable a horse to tuck his feet under easily.

Stand alongside his leg (in this case the left rear) and slide your left hand down his lower leg and lean slightly against him; he should lift his leg. Immediately hold him under his hoof with your right hand. Then, place your left hand under the fetlock joint from the front of his leg. His leg is now resting in your hands and is supported by your left forearm and upper arm. This four-point support is especially helpful if you are working on a large horse. Note that my right upper arm is against the inside of my right knee. This position gives both partners a lot of support. You should adjust your foot position to take a fairly wide stance, especially if your horse has long legs, this is so that you may proceed from a foot rotation to a leg rotation and stretch.

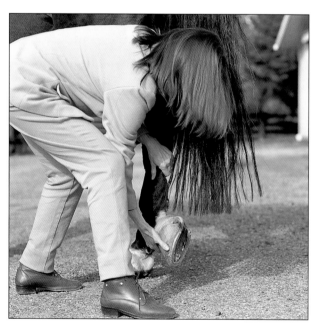
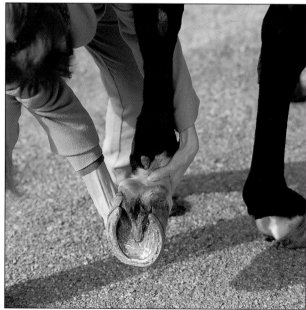

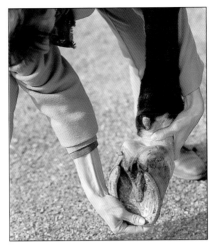
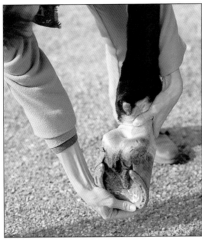
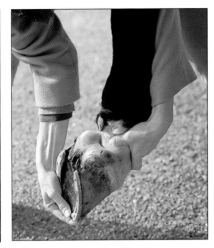

Take hold of the tip of his hoof and rotate it slowly in a full range of motion, or as full as the condition of the joint will allow. You will not be able to move your body as for the front foot rotation, so try to connect the movement to your center and go slowly. You may rotate in either or both directions, although one or the other may seem more harmonious to you, in which case, just rotate in that direction.

Foot stretch

From the basic rotation, stretch the front of his foot to the fetlock joint by lifting his toe *(below left)*. Hold for several seconds. Release the stretch and place the thumb of your working hand on one of the heel bulbs and press downward to stretch the rear portion of his foot *(below right)*. Then, place your thumb on the other bulb and repeat. Working on one heel bulb at a time helps you to become comfortable with holding the leg off the ground while stretching this tiny section. It also makes it easier if you have small hands and the horse has a large foot. If, however, you can cope with using both thumbs simultaneously, it is desirable because it creates an even stretch to the foot.

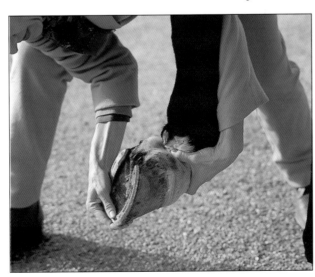
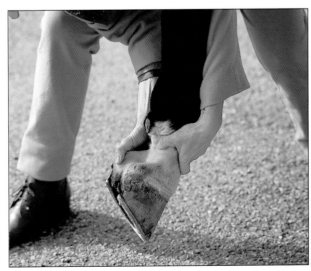

Alternative stretch and rotation position

This is a nice technique for horses who do not yet trust you while you are holding their legs off the ground. It is also good if you have a tired back from other activities.

Place his toe on the ground by bending and taking the leg with you; hold the fetlock joint *(left)*. Simultaneously push the rear of the hoof downward (away from his body), and pull the fetlock forward (toward the front of his body) *(top right)*. Hold this position for several seconds. Then place your hands on the sides of the hoof and rotate his foot with his toe on the ground *(bottom right)*.

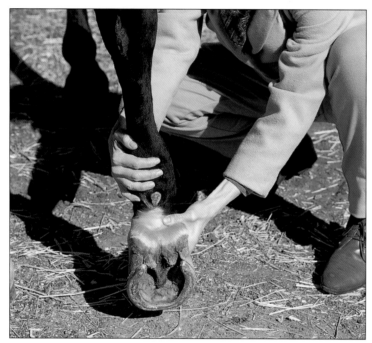
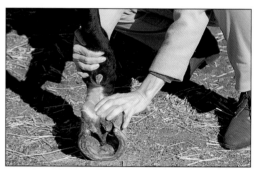
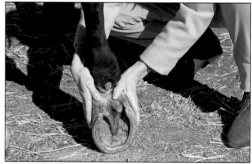

BACK LEG ROTATION AND REARWARD STRETCH

These movements are wonderful for horses with tight backs as they have a positive effect on the back as well as the leg through the hindquarters. All horses will benefit from these techniques and they are especially good for horses who are asked for collected movement. Jumpers appreciate them as well. Remember that smaller rotations will help you feel the condition of the joint, larger ones the condition of the muscles. The rearward stretch will stretch the Stomach Meridian as well as the muscles of the hindquarters and back.

Take a very wide stance and pick up your horse's leg (in this case the right) as previously explained in the section on foot rotation (*see* page 96). Hold your left hand under his hoof, which is raised only slightly off the ground to ensure that there is no compression of the muscles of his hindquarters. Place your right hand at the front of his leg, just below the fetlock joint. His leg is contacting your upper arm and forearm, as explained in the section on foot rotation. Your left upper arm may rest against the inside of your thigh. Your left leg should be well behind him and, of course, slightly to the side of his body. Begin to move your body, taking his leg with you, in small circles, in either or both directions. His leg is directly under him. *(Top left)* Continue rotating as you begin to lean into your left leg and take his leg along a little rearward *(top right)*. Keep rotating as you lean more into your left leg to create a full stretch *(bottom left and right)*. You have now stopped rotating and are supporting his leg from your center, your hands and your arm. If you feel he wants to stretch further you must adjust the position of your feet by moving them along a few inches in the direction of the stretch. If he is very clever and working with you, he will lean forward to create his own stretch, which is ideal. Hold this position for several seconds. Be especially sensitive to any resistance or hesitation on his part and always take his leg to a neutral position just before he takes it himself. To bring his foot under him again, you must shift your weight into your rear leg, bend your knees, and return his foot to the ground, resting on its toe. Or, you may continue holding his leg and proceed to the next technique, which flows nicely from this one.

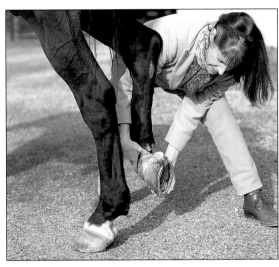
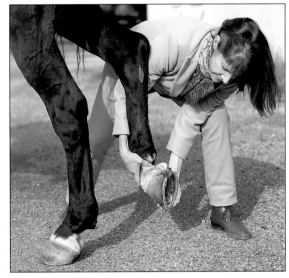
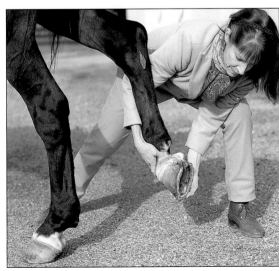
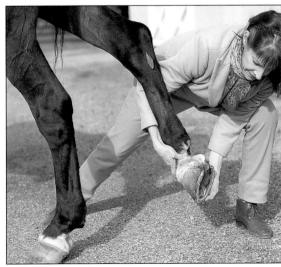

FORWARD STRETCH

This technique will stretch his hamstring muscles as well as the Bladder Meridian in his leg. It is especially helpful for horses who are not tracking up because of tightness. Never force or pull the leg, just use your body to support it. When doing any of these techniques properly, you will feel in your own body the condition of his.

From the rearward stretch position, continue to the forward stretch. Shift your weight into your right leg by bending the right knee and straightening your left leg *(top left)*. Adjust the position of your hands to grasp his leg from the back. In this case, your left hand holds from the outside, the right hand holds from the inside. Your hands should be separated by several inches to give him maximum support. *(Center left.)* This will also help you determine the degree of flexibility or resistance of the stretch. Walk backwards slowly, staying directly alongside his body, taking his leg with you toward his front foot. As you are walking rearward, you are dropping your center by bending your knees. Feel the leg stretch as you lean rearward into your hips, which are nearly on the ground. Hold his leg here for several seconds, always staying sensitive to his needs and coming out of the stretch before he becomes insecure. *(Center right and bottom left.)* To come out of the stretch, shift your weight into your left leg and begin to stand up, taking his leg with you but keeping his foot close to the ground. Take it rearward until it is alongside the other leg and place the foot on the ground by bending your knees and placing the foot on its toe. *(Bottom right.)* You may jiggle the leg again.

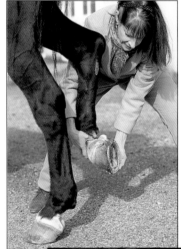

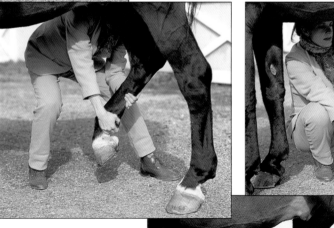

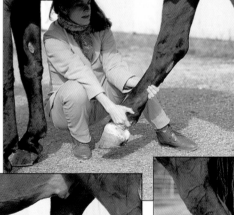

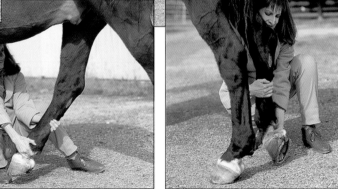

Optional   If you are feeling strong and energetic, before returning your horse's foot to the ground, take it again into the rearward stretch position, recreating your position of a wide stance and leaning your body to stretch his leg. For horses who step to the outside or inside of their front hoof print, I may repeat this rearward and forward sequence several times, thereby patterning their bodies and minds to this more balanced movement.

BACK LEG LIFT AND RELEASE

This is a good technique for horses with extremely tight hindquarters. If you still need to do more after the previous movements, try this one. I also find it helpful for horses whose movement through the quarters is unbalanced when viewed from the back at the walk. Sometimes one hip drops down more then the other. The side that does not have as much movement and stays higher is usually the tighter (more jitsu) side. Work on this side only since this is a sedation technique.

Pick up the leg and hold it off the ground slightly keeping your knees bent. Straighten your legs, taking the leg straight up. The fetlock, hock, and stifle will flex and the muscles in the hindquarters will compress. Hold the leg in this position for two or three seconds, then release it straight down without putting it on the ground. Repeat several times. Then, take it toward the ground in a slightly rearward position a few times. Then lift and release in the first position, about five or six lifts and releases in all. Place his toe on the ground and jiggle. You may wish to have someone walk him so that you may observe a more balanced movement.

If he is at all uncomfortable balancing on the other leg, put his leg down immediately and leave the exercise until another time.

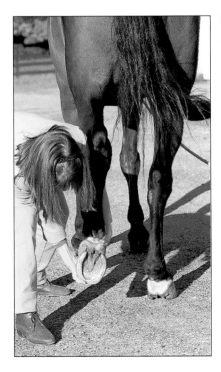
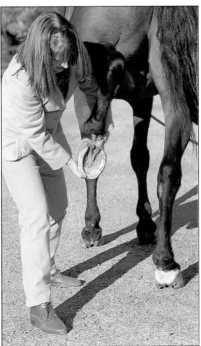
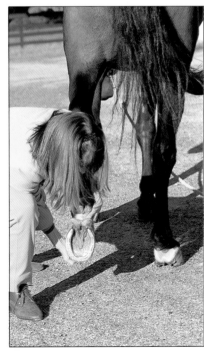

MERIDIAN STRETCHES

Here are a few stretches that will specifically stretch meridians. They are variations on the stretches you have done in the previous section. You may do them before or after actually working on the meridians. Stretching meridians activates the energy in them and may help to increase energy flow. Meridian stretches are particularly good when you have worked on a meridian, and found it tight and jitsu. Therefore, stretching is actually a sedation technique. Big prolonged stretches should not be done on horses whose energy is depleted.

Gall Bladder Meridian stretch

Take the leg into a rearward stretch position and, as you hold it there, take it toward the other leg. You will be almost crossing the leg behind the other leg; this will stretch the Gall Bladder Meridian, which is on the outside of the leg. (Stretching the leg directly rearward will stretch the Stomach Meridian.)

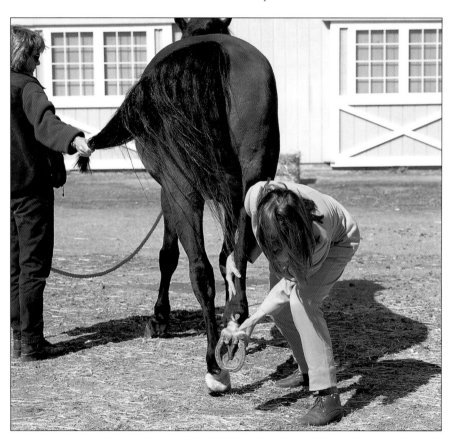

Yin meridians stretch – Kidney, Liver, and Spleen Meridians

This is a general stretch for the yin meridians, which may be altered slightly to specifically access each one individually. Pick up the leg and stretch it slightly out to the side. Taking it to the side and slightly forward (only a few inches) will stretch the Kidney Meridian. Taking it directly out to the side will stretch the Spleen Meridian. Taking it out to the side and slightly rearward (only a few inches) will stretch the Liver Meridian.

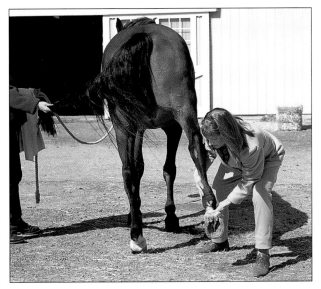 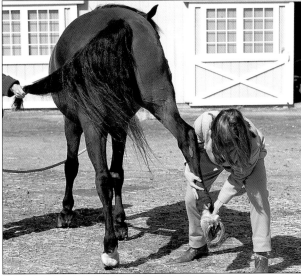

As you hold the leg several seconds in these positions, concentrate on feeling any restriction in energy flow. Put the leg down immediately if your horse is at all resistant or feeling insecure in any of these positions. Remember that he may be uncomfortable supporting himself on the other leg.

Alternative Kidney Meridian stretch

Take the leg toward the front hoof, only this time take it slightly outward. Hold several seconds. The position where the rear foot points directly toward the front hoof stretches the Bladder Meridian.

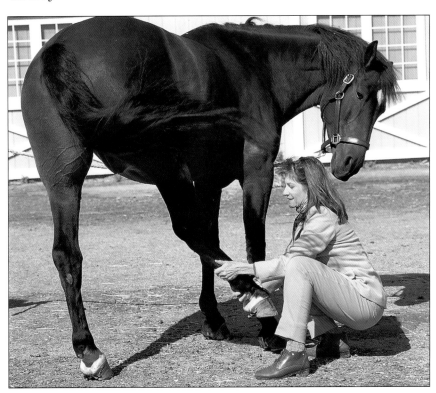

MERIDIAN WORK

As with the front legs, you must adjust your angles so that your body leans directly toward or directly away from the meridian on which you are working. Always press these points vertically to the surface of the skin. Do not slide on the skin. You may work on points at intervals of two or three inches apart, or closer together, or several inches apart. You must trust your instincts and always work according to the needs of your horse.

For a detailed reference to each of the following meridians, *see* Meridian Locations.

Bladder Meridian

As a continuation of working the Bladder Meridian from the section for the back and hindquarters (*see* pages 64–71) continue down the leg as shown. Place your inside hand (this is your supporting hand) around his leg just above the hock and place your fingertips, which are close together, directly in the meridian. Your working hand holds from the outside. Begin with your hands close together and proceed downward with your working hand. You will achieve pressure by leaning your body rearward each time your working hand contacts the next point along the meridian line. When your hands get too far apart, move your supporting hand downward, perhaps below the hock this time, and continue down the leg.

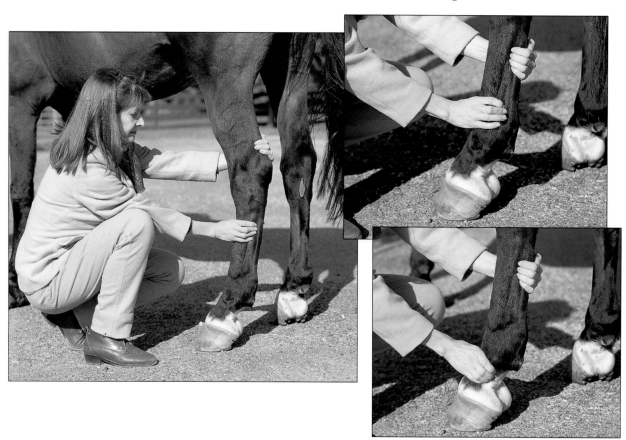

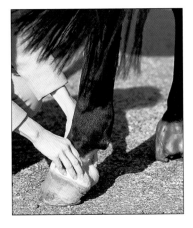

Optional   Place the leg in a stretch position by lifting it and placing the foot on the ground slightly nearer the front foot. This will create a slight stretch that, with a horse who is tight in this area, may be beneficial. You should note that the meridian will feel even tighter because of the position of the leg.

Working on the foot
Having finished the Bladder Meridian, press all the points around the foot, concentrating on the end point of the meridian. To work the last point on the Bladder Meridian, hold firmly with your thumb for several seconds.

Note   Working on the foot in this way is important when finishing work on all meridians.

Stomach Meridian

Place your supporting palm somewhere on the upper leg on the Stomach Meridian (you may wish to use Stomach 36 [*see* Point Location Charts]). You may also use the thumb of the supporting hand. Move down the meridian toward the foot with your working hand. Do this by leaning your body toward the leg to achieve vertical pressure. As your hands become too far apart, move your supporting hand down the leg, still keeping it on the meridian *(below, far right)*. The new position of your working hand may be on a point or area that felt kyo to your touch when you did the all-over stroking. Work this meridian all the way down to the foot.

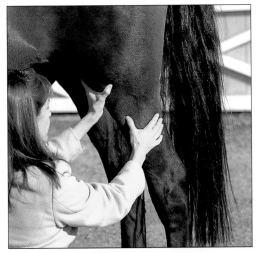

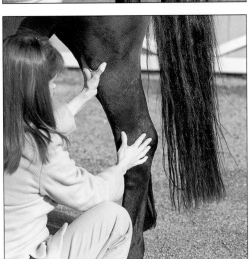

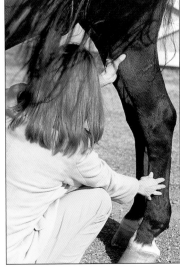

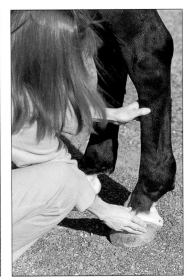

Yin meridians of the back leg

The yin meridians of the back leg are the Kidney, Liver, and Spleen Meridians. This is a guideline for working on any of these meridians. Remember that yin meridians are more protected, being on the inside parts of the horse's body, and are more sensitive. They should be treated with more tenderness than the yang meridians.

Position your body facing toward the leg you are working on. Place the fingertips of your supporting hand high up on the inside of the leg and the fingertips of your working hand just below. Work down the meridian toward the foot in small increments. The pressure is achieved by leaning your body rearward. When your hands get too far apart, move the supporting hand further down the leg, still in the meridian, and continue down to the foot. Your supporting hand may move three times according to the length of the leg you are working on.

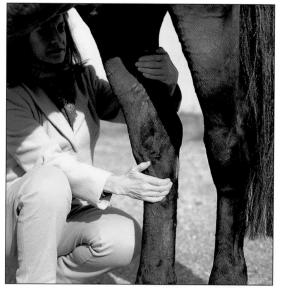
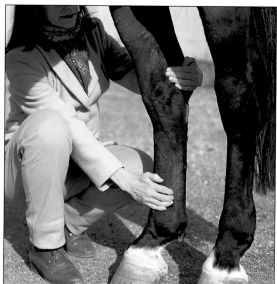
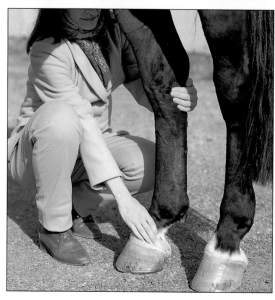

Percussion Technique

This is a valuable technique for loosening the muscles and bringing circulation to areas of big muscle groups. It is a technique from the modality of Swedish massage. I like it because it wakes up the sleepy horse as well as relaxing the overly excited horse. It is a technique that brings awareness of muscle tension or pain to both the horse and practitioner while it releases muscle tension. It should be used after you have completed your other techniques such as meridian work, rotations, and stretching. This is a sedation technique and therefore should not be used on horses who are extremely tired, or recovering from illness or surgery. Avoid sensitive areas, and areas of swelling or soreness.

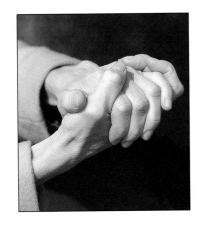

Clasp your hands and create a pocket of air between your palms. This is important, as this pocket of air will be absorbing some of the impact as you rhythmically strike and bounce your hands off your horse's body. Without actually making contact, practice moving your hands from the wrists. If you are right handed, most of the wrist movement will be initiated from the right wrist, although the left wrist will move a bit as well. The speed of the movement is about twice per second. Now, practice on yourself by bouncing the back of your hand off your own thigh. If your wrists are relaxed, you should hear a whoosh of the air caught between your palms with each contact. Your hands should bounce off your leg each time. This is a loose movement from your wrists that results in a firm contact on the body. Practice changing speed as well as the amount of pressure as you work on your own leg before you apply this technique to your horse. It is also a good idea to try this technique with a friend. Bend over from the waist and let your body dangle, your arms relaxed loosely toward the floor. Have your friend work on the muscles along the sides of your spine and buttocks, as well as down the sides and back of your legs. Have them vary the speed and amount of pressure. Try it on your friend as well and ask for feedback.

I particularly like this technique for the muscles of the hindquarters. I occasionally use it on the muscles alongside the spine or on the sides of the neck of certain horses. These horses are very well muscled and strong, and usually yang types (*see* page 231). Do not practice this technique on a yin type horse (*see* page 230) as they will find it disturbing and perhaps painful. As you work on the large muscles, you should see them moving in response to your work. This technique moves muscles and in a well-balanced horse you should see a nice undulation in response to percussion.

As a variation, practice percussion without actually removing your hands from the body. This means you are pulsing your hands rather than striking the body. I only do this variation on the muscles of the hindquarters.

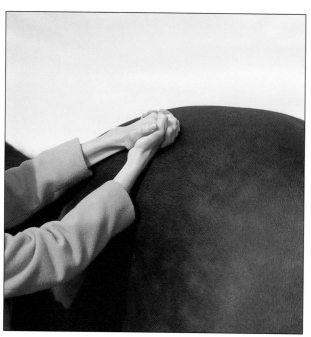
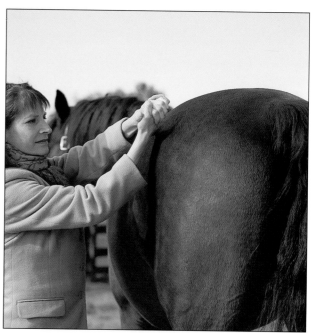
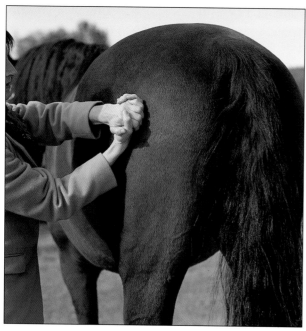
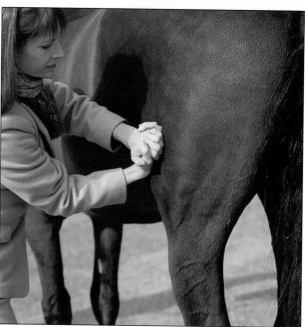

The Tail

The tail is a mobile and expressive part of the spine. It is a part of the horse's body from which we can understand how he is feeling about himself and what he is doing. It is well known that a horse with a clamped tail may be feeling insecure and a horse who is wringing and swishing his tail during work is decidedly not happy with his activity, or in pain. I touch the tail for a variety of reasons and, as with most shiatsu techniques, diagnosis is treatment and treatment is diagnosis. As you work on the tail, you may notice tightness when you move it from side to side. You may relate this to the side of his back that was tighter as you worked along his Bladder Meridian. Working on the tail will promote flexibility and awareness in the tail as well as the rest of the vertebrae of the spine. It is said that the last vertebra of the body relates to the first vertebra. Therefore, working on the tail may have an effect on the neck, and vice versa. This is very useful because some horses may object to having their necks worked on. Also remember that working on any area of a meridian will affect the energy throughout the entire meridian.

Most horses welcome work on the tail, although a mare in season may not be a candidate until she is out of season. These techniques will help the horse develop awareness of his tail as well as improved tail carriage. He will become aware of how his tail really feels and how much it can move and that it is an important part of his spine and of the flowing balanced movement of his body. If he has never been touched so extensively on his tail he will really seem to be thinking about what he is feeling.

During your preliminary observation of the horse at the walk before you begin your session, remember to look at the tail and notice if it is carried off to one side, or if it is clamped down. These are signs of possible tightness and pain in the back, or the neck, or both. Work on the tail in the middle of the session or towards the end when the horse is relaxed. It is a good technique to incorporate into the session after working on the back and rear legs. You may want to do the beginning tail techniques in the middle of your session, and finish the tail near the end of your session.

When working on the tail, work your hands toward it from whatever previous technique you use so as not to surprise him, rather than just suddenly touching his tail, which will cause suspicion and clamping. Some horses turn around and look at me when I first touch their tails. I look back and tell them it is me and not to worry. Always be aware of their body language as you work on this area. Look at their ears which should be angled back to show they are listening to you, but not pinned back. If they pin back their ears, let go of the tail and walk to the head, keeping hand contact as you go, and reassure them, relax them, and try again. There is always tomorrow. I only do the tail work on horses who are very relaxed and trustworthy. If you have any doubt about working on the tail of a particular horse, do not do it. Wait until another day and try again, introducing the techniques gradually. Each horse takes a different amount of time to learn how to receive shiatsu, as each person takes a different amount of time to learn to give it.

STROKING THE TAIL

This beginning technique will give your horse time to become accustomed to having his tail touched. It will also give you the opportunity to get all the tail hair gathered out of the way so you will not be pulling hairs inadvertently. It will help you to understand something of his personality as well. If he is holding his tail against his body, he may be insecure about having his tail touched, or just generally insecure. Some horses have tails that feel too relaxed and floppy in your hands. These tails seem to be lacking energy and not to be connected with the energy of the rest of the spine. This may be the result of an injury to the tail or simply indicates a lack of energy or awareness of the tail.

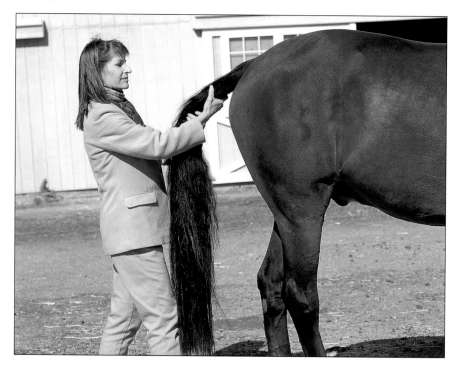

Gently lift the tail away from his body and begin stroking from underneath with alternating hands. Lean your body slightly rearward with each movement of your hands to create smooth continuity. Repeat this technique until the tail feels relaxed in your hands. The horse may even begin to lower his head. This is not a pulling technique.

WALKING THE TAIL

This technique will reconfirm any tightness in his back that you felt when working on the Bladder Meridian. Do it slowly and with concentration and awareness.

Holding the tail with the hand position of the previous technique, begin to walk toward his hindquarters, taking the tail with you. As you walk, adjust the position of your hands so that both hands are across the top of the tail. The hands should be about ten inches apart. Drape the tail along the horse's body, letting it conform to the shape of the hindquarters. Take care that there is no compression at the top of the tail on the side that you are on. If there is, place the tail lower on the hindquarters. Do not pull, just hold the tail here for several seconds to observe the degree of flexibility and let your horse feel the contact of his tail on his body. Then, walk the tail to the other side as you adjust your hands so that they are both across the top of the tail by the time you drape it across his body on the other side. Repeat this walking from side to side at least three times on each side.

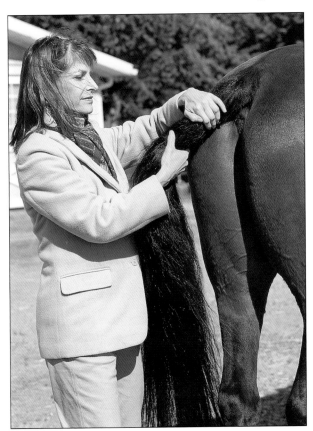
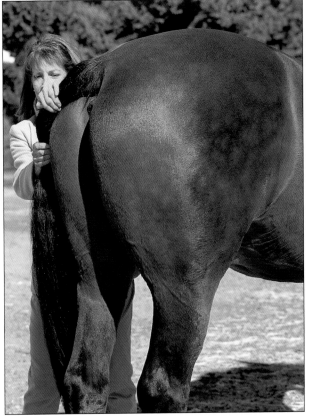

ROTATING THE DOCK

The dock is the connection between the lumbar vertebrae and the vertebrae of the tail. I feel it is an important area for increasing awareness and energy flow, as well as increased flexibility.

Place both hands under the tail as high up and close together as possible. Stand far enough away from him so that your elbows are softly bent. Hold the tail firmly but do not grab or squeeze it. Begin moving the tail in a circular motion slowly, exploring its range of motion. Do not pull it toward you, but do not push it toward his back either. Rotate in either or both directions.

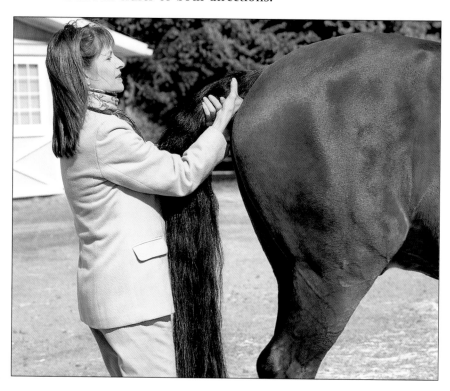

INDIVIDUAL ROTATION OF VERTEBRAE

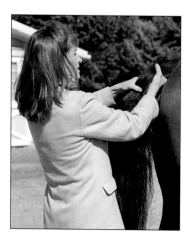

This technique will completely exercise his tail vertebrae. It will help you understand the condition of all the joints, and give him a sense of the extent of the movement his tail is capable of. You may notice that there is much less movement toward the end of the tail bones than at the beginning. Never force these rotations. You may rotate in either or both directions. Go very slowly. Each rotation should take at least five seconds to complete.

Begin with your supporting hand at the top of the tail, holding it underneath. Your working hand will be positioned directly below the supporting hand and may hold from underneath, on top or the side of the tail, whichever you find more comfortable. The supporting hand does not move during the rotation. Moving from your center, and using your working hand to create the movement, begin to rotate the first vertebra, exploring its range of motion. Rotate three or four times until you rotate in the largest circle the tail will trace comfortably. This movement comes from moving your body, not just your hands. To move to the next vertebra, lean rearward, and slide both hands down. You may feel the side of the index finger of the supporting hand slip into the space between the vertebrae. This is desirable, as you will know that you have gone down the tail in an increment of one tail bone. You will be standing further and further away from your horse as you come to the end of the tail.

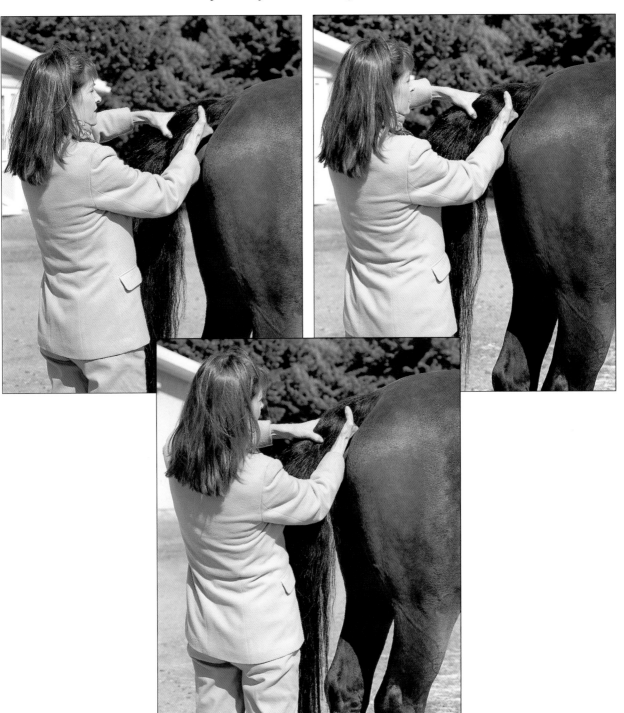

TAIL LIFT

This exercise will improve awareness for both the horse and the practitioner: for the horse, awareness that his tail can arc section by section thus improving tail carriage; for the practitioner, awareness of the flexibility of each section of the tail. Go slowly, as usual, with your attention on your horse's response.

Place your supporting hand under the tail close to its top. Place your working hand just below it and across the upper part of the tail. Your hands will stay close together throughout this technique. Push upward only slightly with your supporting hand and hold. Using your working hand, which is on top of the tail, draw it downward, creating a soft arc in the tail. This is a gentle subtle movement. Hold the position for about three to five seconds. Proceed to the next segment by leaning slightly rearward and sliding your hands along until you feel the side of the index finger of the supporting hand slip into the next space between the vertebrae. Work down the tail in this way, moving further away from your horse. You will notice that the end of the tail probably will not move so only do the places that move effortlessly.

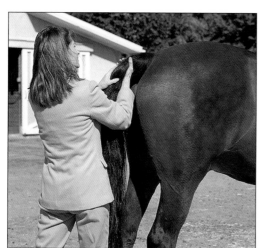

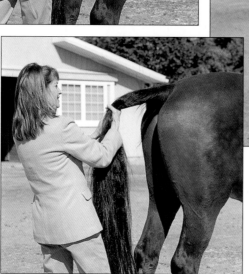

FULL STRETCH

Hold your hands underneath the tail with the upper hand placed about one third of the way down from the top and the lower hand two thirds of the way down. Both hands must be holding bones. Make sure your horse is standing fairly evenly on all four feet, with his head forward if possible. Position yourself with one foot at least twelve to fifteen inches behind you. The knee of the back foot will bend as you drop your weight into the foot and your hip. Slowly begin to lean rearward. You will be dropping your weight into your hip, lower body and your back foot. The tail position is a natural one, not held up or pulled downward from the body. The tail bones are in natural alignment with his spine. Keep leaning to the maximum and wait for your horse to stretch away from you. He may be so relaxed and leaning forward to such an extent that you will have difficulty maintaining your position. Try to support him as he stretches his entire spine all the way to his neck. He should lower his head. If he looks around at you, reassure him and ask him to straighten his head. Try to hold this stretch for at least ten seconds. Your bodies should be in complete harmony during this stretch even though you are standing away from him. To come out of this stretch (your back will get a nice stretch as well) gradually pull yourself toward him as you shift your weight to your forward foot. This slow release is important. Let go of his tail, walk to his head and observe his demeanor for a moment. Compliment him on his cooperation.

If you hear little cracking sounds as you stretch do not be concerned. It is merely the release of fluid in the joints and is of no concern.

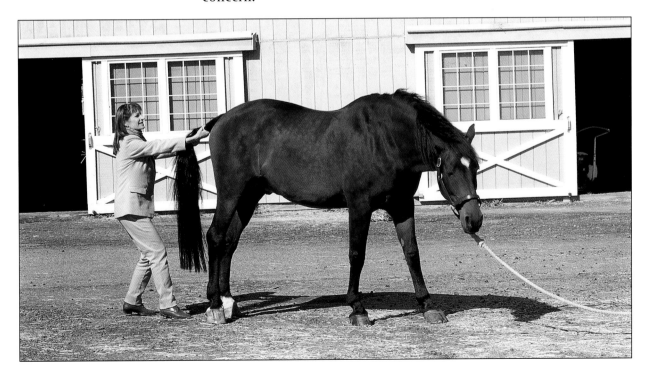

The Neck

Neck work is often done at the end of the session. Many horses are sensitive in this area and may not allow you to do much, especially during the first few tries. Be extremely patient, go slowly and gradually. Your horse needs to learn these techniques along with you. Neck work may help misaligned vertebrae find their proper place; however, we are not actively trying to adjust the neck. When energy is in balance, bones may naturally find their proper position. If you suspect misaligned neck vertebrae, especially after you have worked on your horse, consult a practitioner with experience in this area.

NECK JIGGLE

Always begin with the jiggling unless you suspect that your horse has a headache. To determine if he is headachy, look into his eyes, look at the expression around his eyes as well as the entire head carriage. His attitude generally will help you to understand how he is feeling.

The jiggling causes his head to rock from side to side while his neck is going in the opposite direction. This may be disturbing to some horses as it feels like a lack of control. If your horse needs to be in control at all times, even when relaxed, he may object to neck jiggling (or jiggling anywhere else on his body).

Start off slowly, setting up the most minor of movements. Carefully observe his expression as you go. The initial placement of your hands on his neck is important also. You may wish to begin with your hands in the center of his neck. If he is happy with this, move your hands to various locations along his crest as you rock, and try to find his favorite place. Always finish with your hands located in his favorite position.

The jiggle

Place your hands side by side in the center of his crest. Your hands mold to the shape of his body and your relaxed fingertips are draped across the far side of his neck. Begin to move your body from your feet all the way up into your hands. You will appear to be rocking forward and back. Go slowly at first until you feel the movement throughout your entire body. This movement should carry through into your horse's body, causing his neck to move and his head to rock gently from side to side. If he likes this, put a bit more energy into your movement. Remember that this is not done from your shoulders, but from your center. If he is not too sure he likes this, diminish your movement or gradually stop and try another time. If he is having a good time and beginning to loosen his head as shown, move your hands from location to location, rocking several times in each location, and making smooth transitions to the next place on his neck. The transition is important and to keep it smooth, try to keep him moving a bit as you move your hands each time. At the end of the technique, gradually stop rocking so that the movement does not stop abruptly. Take a moment to observe his reaction to the jiggling.

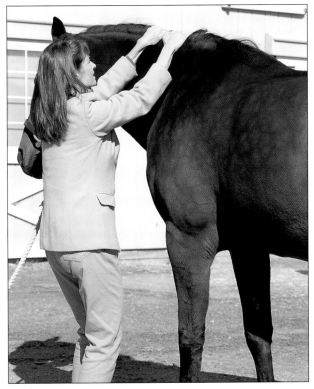

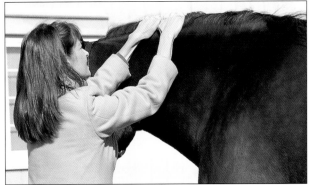

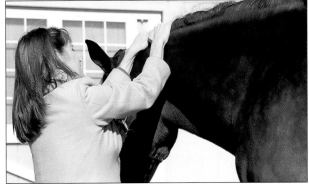

NECK MERIDIANS

There are six meridians in the neck and each is bilateral. They are the Stomach, Large Intestine, Small Intestine, Triple Heater, Gall Bladder and Bladder Meridians. For a detailed reference to each of these meridians, *see* Meridian Locations. For general neck work you may choose to work areas rather than specific meridians. The following photographs show me working by area, although you may say that I am working either the Triple Heater or Small Intestine Meridians in the central area, the Bladder or Gall Bladder Meridians in the upper portion of the neck and the Stomach or Large Intestine Meridians in the lower portion. If you know your horse has the need for particular meridian work, use these techniques as guidelines. The neck is a good area to feel a lot of energy movement, so take your time and stay keenly aware of your horse's reactions. Your all-over stroking may have taught you that one side of his neck would be the more comfortable to begin on. Always start on the easier side. This applies to the stretching techniques as well. Always stretch the more flexible side first.

The neck techniques are demonstrated here in a logical progression of assessing and addressing the neck for increased comfort, awareness and, if needed, flexibility. The jiggling relaxes him and shows you his level of security and the meridian work gets his energy moving and helps you both become aware of any imbalances in energy and muscle tightness. This way, you will know exactly the amount of movement you can expect before you actually move his neck and head. Your horse will be secure and relaxed if you always proceed in a logical sequence, each technique preparing the way for the next, and each ensuing technique a natural progression from the previous one.

THREE LINES WITH THE NECK IN A NEUTRAL POSITION

Center line

Place your working hand on his neck with your opposite foot slightly behind you. Your supporting hand is on the same location on the opposite side of his neck. Lean from your body to gradually apply pressure into your working hand's palm heel. Your supporting hand presses toward your working hand, using the entire palm's surface. This will keep his head in a neutral position. Hold this point for several seconds or until you feel some energy response from your horse. Gradually release the pressure and, without lifting your hand off the neck, lean into the next point, a couple of inches from the first location. Your supporting hand has also moved along on the far side. Work this way toward the shoulder either increasing or decreasing pressure to ensure his comfort and trust. You may do a bit of jiggling if you like before proceeding to the next technique.

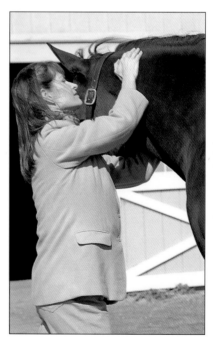
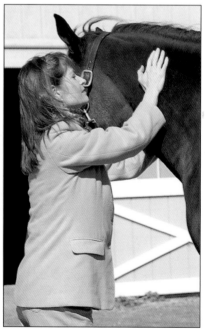
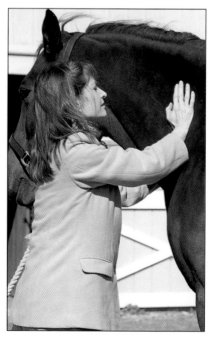

Top line

Place the palm of your working hand in the muscle just below the crest, with the rest of your hand in contact and molding to him. Your opposite foot is slightly behind you. Your supporting hand is on the far side of his neck in the area of the Stomach and Large Intestine Meridians. The direction of pressure of your working hand is always vertical to the surface you are working on. In the case of his upper neck, for the first few points you will be pressing downward, to accommodate his anatomy in this area. Your supporting hand will be pressing upward. The hands will move along together, sandwiching his neck as you move from beginning to end. For you to create the downward pressure on the first few points, let your knees bend and feel your center dropping downward. Always keep his neck in a neutral position for this technique. As he relaxes and lowers his head, you will have to adjust your body posture to accommodate his.

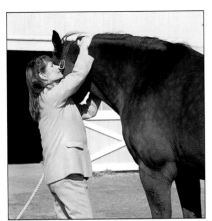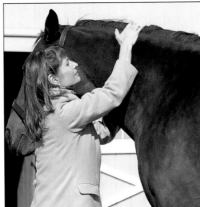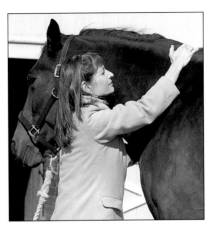

Bottom line

Apply your working hand to the area under his neck and your supporting hand on the far side in the area of the Bladder Meridian. To achieve pressure, stand with the foot opposite to the working hand slightly behind you, with both knees slightly bent. Straighten your knees a little, which will assist in creating upward pressure to the neck with your working palm. The supporting hand on the far side is pressing downward, again creating a sandwich effect. Begin on the upper neck and proceed toward the shoulder, working in small increments.

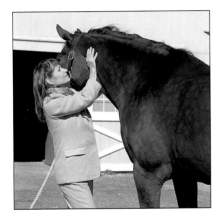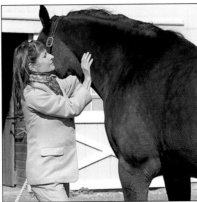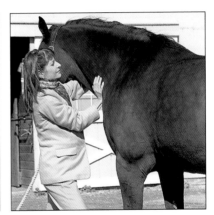

BE FLEXIBLE IN YOUR NECK PROCEDURE

If your horse suddenly objects and expresses pain, go back to the previous area where he felt comfortable, talk to him, and encourage him to relax his neck by squatting in front of him for a moment. Run your hand lightly across the area to check for any heat, swelling, fullness or emptiness in the area where he feels pain. You may wish to temporarily discontinue the neck work and proceed to the shoulders or back, then come back to the neck later in the treatment. Or you may work as follows.

In the case of heat (where there is no broken skin), swelling (not from any known source) or feeling of excessive energy, work on the meridian that passes through that area, avoiding the location of specific pain. Do this two or three times and check again to determine if the pain has disappeared. If not, work on the rest of the meridian throughout his body, both sides, and check his neck again. It may be that there is no evidence of the sensitivity you first detected. You may now continue with neck work. If there is still discomfort after a few days and the quality of his rest and work is adversely affected, consult your vet.

INCREMENTAL NECK WORK

This technique is a valuable learning tool for you both. It creates awareness of the individual vertebrae of the neck and their independent movement. It also helps to determine the exact location of any dislocation in alignment. The movement is very small as it is not a stretching technique; this is important to note while moving the neck.

It is an exercise in awareness as a precursor to stretching. The horse becomes aware of the fact that he has sections of his neck that move to create the smooth movement of the entire neck. He may learn from this exercise that his neck only hurts in one place rather than the entire neck and be more willing to let you work on the nonpainful places if he had previously been reluctant to let you do any meridian work at all on his neck. The head only moves a few inches each time your hand moves to the next position along the neck. After each movement, the head is returned to a neutral position.

Place your supporting hand across his nose, or on his far-side cheek. Your working hand is near the top of his neck, in the large muscle. The foot opposite to the working hand is slightly behind you. *(Opposite top.)* Lean gradually into the palm of the working hand with gentle pressure. By turning your body in a twisting motion toward his head, turn his head a few inches toward you. *(Opposite bottom.)* Hold him in this position for a few seconds before returning his head to a neutral position. Note that you are not pulling his head with your hand, rather causing it to move by the turning motion of your entire body. Proceed down the entire length of the neck in this way, moving your hand to about seven or eight positions along the neck. Do both sides. If he objects to any area, always go back to the previously accepted technique. Avoid twisting his head; keep his head vertical.

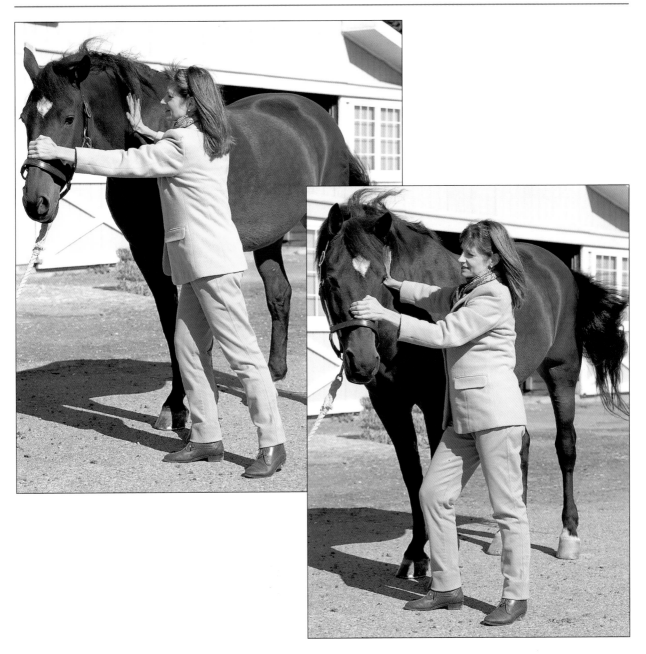

NECK STRETCH TO EACH SIDE

By now you have determined exactly how far and with what degree of comfort your horse will be able to stretch his neck to the side with your assistance. This is important, for now you may proceed to this stretch with his complete confidence and trust *(see photos on page 122)*.

This stretch is large and wide and stretches both sides of the neck. Keep in mind that you do not want to compress one side while stretching the other. A horse may be able to easily scratch an itch on his hindquarters by himself but the execution of an assisted stretch may be difficult. This stretch is done slowly and with control, and the release back to the neutral position is also done slowly and methodically.

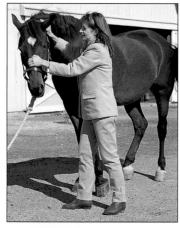

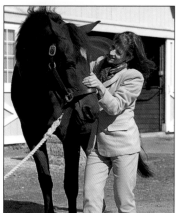

Your body is in the same position as in the previous exercise. Start by placing your hands in the same position as previously shown. Your hand will move down his neck in small increments without returning his head to the neutral position each time. Each time your hand moves down the neck, his head moves around you in a wide arc. Bring the head around your body, rather than tightly toward his shoulder. You may wish to establish eye contact as you encourage him to bring his head around, and pull him with your eyes. Use your instincts keenly to be aware of any tightness or insecurity on his part. If he is insecure, reassure him without moving his head further, then proceed only if he is relaxed. If he is tight, release the stretch slightly and then continue, or place his head in a completely neutral position and try again. Try to keep his head from twisting around. Avoid letting him take his head away from you and swinging it around on his own. Always use your entire body to bring his head around you, rather than only pulling with your arms. Working in this way, you will sense any tightness or discomfort because you are working with him, not forcing him. You use your energy to move his energy and create harmony between you.

This technique may be used as a range-of-motion exercise, rather than a stretch. Some horses actually do not need stretching. However, range-of-motion exercises will keep them supple, aware of their bodies and less prone to injury. You will have a much better understanding of their bodies, as well as your own. You may stretch each side more than once, always starting and finishing on the easier side.

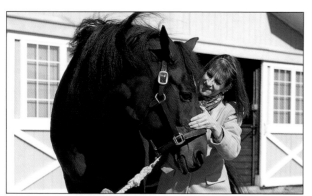

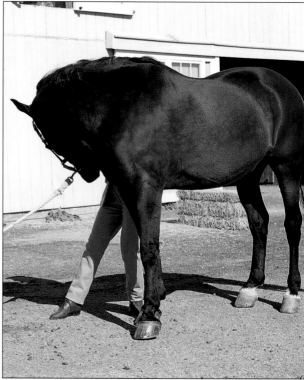

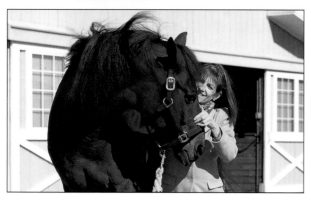

ALTERNATIVE SIDE STRETCH

Your size in relation to your horse's size is important for this alternative side stretch. If you are able to make contact with his neck with your head and shoulders, it will work for you. Do this if your horse is at all reluctant to do the previous stretch. It is an alternative but is not meant to replace the full, supported stretch previously explained.

Take hold of his withers with one hand and with the other reach under his chin and across his nose, or just hold his far cheek with your palm. With the back of your head or shoulders in supportive contact with his neck, bend him around your body. This technique feels like a big hug and should feel especially good for both of you. Hold this position for several seconds and, with support, return his head to its neutral position. Avoid having your head positioned under his neck or head for obvious safety reasons.

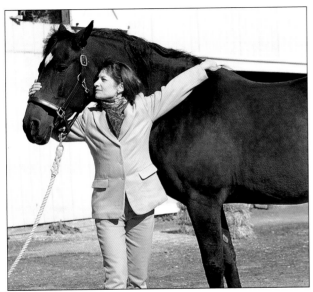
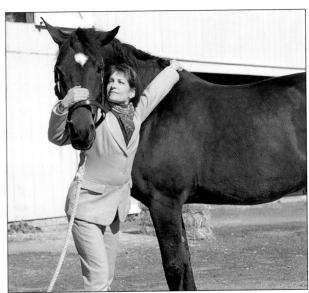
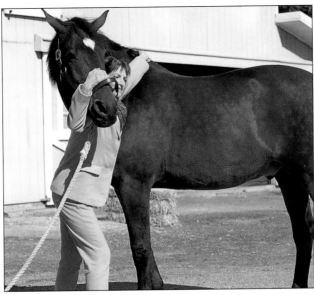

RELEASING TENSION OF THE POLL AREA

This is a great technique for helping horses with headaches. They may not appear to appreciate it immediately, so just practice the initial holding position without any side to side movement. Just encourage him to lower his head while applying gentle but steady pressure behind his ears as shown below. The Bladder and Gall Bladder Meridian points your hand will fall into are especially effective for head, eye, and neck tension.

Place your palm heel on one side of your horse's neck and your four fingers (which are touching each other) on his neck directly on the poll area. Your other hand is across his nose. By gradually dropping your center (lowering your knees if necessary), your horse may begin to lower his head. Hold him in this relaxed position while applying a bit more pressure to the poll. This is a sort of squeezing feeling. Stay in this position for as long as he likes, which may be several minutes. You may then try some movement, which will be a gentle rocking to each side (only an inch or two at first). This is achieved by using the hand that is across his nose to guide the movement. If he is comfortable and happy, you may wish to increase the rocking a bit more, but avoid swinging his head for too long (thirty seconds should be the maximum). Gradually decrease the movement to stillness and hold for several seconds before proceeding to another technique.

You may also use this position to rock his nose downward. Using the hand that is across his nose, bob his chin an inch or two toward his chest a few times, releasing it to whatever position he takes. Do this several times, possibly increasing the movement if he is comfortable and happy.

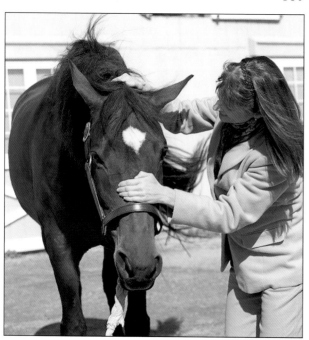
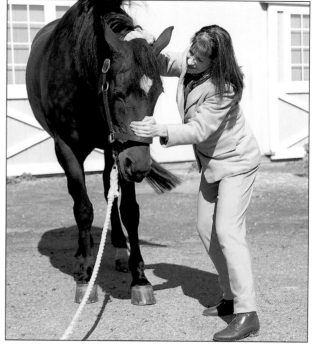

In addition, you may alter the position of the hand that is on the poll. Instead of holding with the palm and four fingers, try holding with the thumb and the middle two fingers. Let your fingers find points in this area where they sink in and feel natural. You will perhaps find kyo points. Avoid holding jitsu points as they will be too sensitive. Perhaps wait until you have worked on him more than once before attempting this variation. Note that the points may be very sensitive, especially on a horse with a headache, or upper neck or lower back problem. They are good diagnostic points for these problems.

To continue releasing the poll, you may, again, incorporate side to side movement. Holding your hand in the same position as described above, behind his ears, place your other hand under his chin, grasping both sides if possible, and not pressing upward. Slowly begin to tilt his head by pulling his nose toward you, holding for a few seconds, then tilting it away from you and holding for a few seconds. Hold just at the point where you feel the slightest muscle tension from his body. Keep your own body relaxed, with your knees soft, as shown. Repeat this side to side tilting a few times. You will not necessarily be trying to increase his range of motion, just exercising this area and helping him become more aware of the possibility of movement in this area. Stay aware of your own body as you develop your techniques. Continue deep, low, abdominal breathing, keep your body soft and flowing, and your face relaxed.

You may now wish to jiggle his neck a bit so that both of you can notice the increased flexibility and ease of his entire neck.

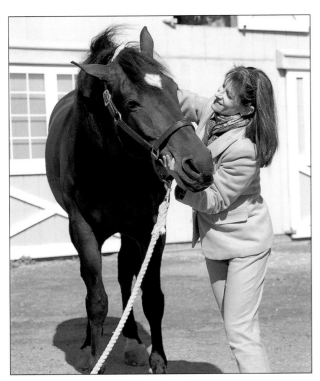
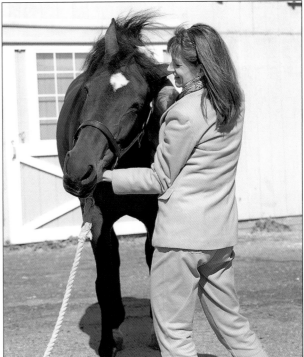

NECK EXTENSION

This exercise may actually teach your horse to lengthen his neck by himself. As with most of these movements, you just happen to be there in a supportive and nonforceful way. The lengthening stretch may relieve long-held neck tension that side to side movements cannot relieve. This is a great technique to do toward the end of your neck work, if you choose to use it.

First, hold his head behind the ears and under his chin. Encourage him to lower his head if he is not already doing so. Lean to the side, taking him with you. You may take up to ten seconds to achieve your maximum position for the stretch. The hand supporting his neck is pressing downward and toward his nose. The hand supporting his chin is pulling directly forward. If someone is near, ask them to observe his neck and let you know when they see physical lengthening.

Notice the gradual progression of stretch as shown in these photos. Also notice that I am not pulling or forcing. Look at my body and understand that I am leaning and taking him with me. At the first (or before the first) point of resistance, stop leaning and just hold to support. Especially smart and cooperative horses will begin to lean rearward after you stop leaning away, to help create more of a stretch for themselves.

This is a wonderful technique that your horse may feel all the way along his back. It will feel very good to you as well because you may be able to completely relax your body as you lean away and let his weight support you completely.

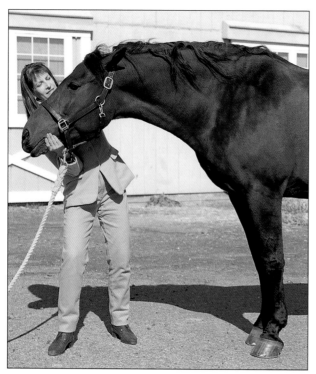
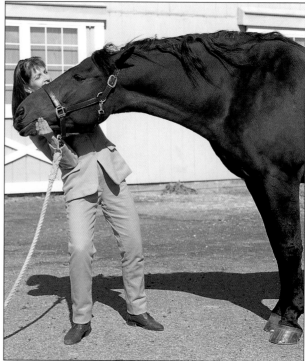

Alternative holding position

For horses who need more support and security during this stretch, try the holding position shown here. The hand on his head remains the same; the hand under his chin goes all the way to the other side of his face. You may hold his face against the side of your body in a soft hug, then lean into your leg furthest from the horse to stretch. Hold him here for as long as he wishes.

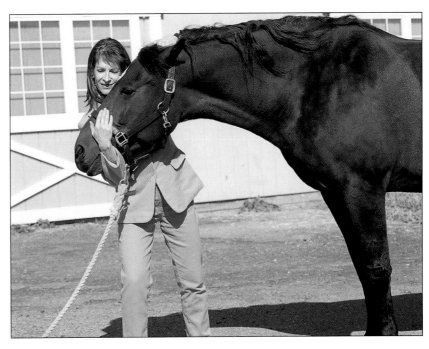

ADDITIONAL LENGTHENING STRETCH POSITION

Avoid this technique on a horse who has the habit of tossing his head. If your horse is very relaxed and cuddly, it will work well for you.

Encourage him to rest his chin on your shoulder. Hold one hand across his nose, well above the nostrils, and the other hand on his head behind his ears as shown. You will have one leg well behind you. Stay in this position for several seconds or until you feel him relax and rest a bit of the weight of his head on your shoulder. The weight on your shoulder should be halfway between your neck and the outside of your shoulder, in your upper trapezious muscle, and should feel as if he is giving you shiatsu in this area. Begin to lean into your rear leg, taking his head with you. At the first point of resistance, stop leaning for a moment to make certain of his comfort and security, then lean a bit further rearward. If he is happy and cooperative, he may begin to lean rearward to increase the stretch. Release the stretch by gradually shifting your weight toward him.

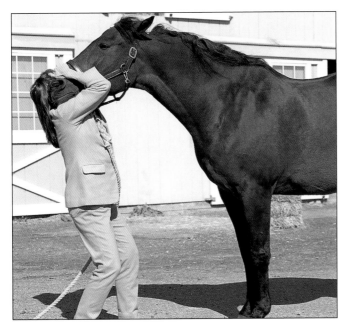

MODIFIED LENGTHENING STRETCH

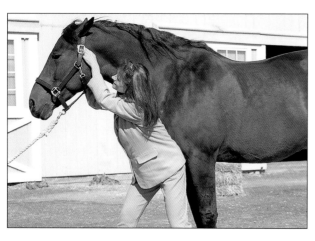

This is another technique where your relative sizes are important. Stand in front of him, facing in the same direction, and fit his chest into the small of your back. You may have to bend your knees a bit to do so. If he is too tall, do not do this variation. Place the index-finger side of your hands behind his cheekbones. Press your hips rearward into his chest while pressing his head forward. This technique calls for some strength in your upper body, since you are becoming a 'human traction machine', which is what I like to call the technique. Try to hold and stretch his neck in this position for several seconds and gradually release. Take good care not to position your head under his neck, rather out to the side as shown.

ADDITIONAL NECK STRETCHING TECHNIQUE

If your horse is reluctant to bend his neck toward you for a stretch and persists in turning his head away from you, you may utilize this movement for a stretch. Place a supporting hand on his neck, and the other across his nose. Press the hand that is on the neck toward you, while gradually guiding his head away from you. Do a minimum stretch, then return his head to the forward position. Next, repeat the movement, while guiding his head a little further around, away from you, and hold it in a stretched position for a few seconds. Repeat two or three times, then move to the other side and try stretching his neck toward you (you will still be stretching his neck in the same direction).

Always stretch the easier side first, never force, be patient, and remember that you are guiding the neck, not pushing it.

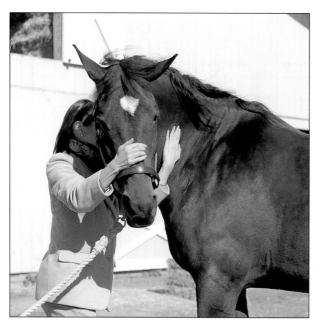

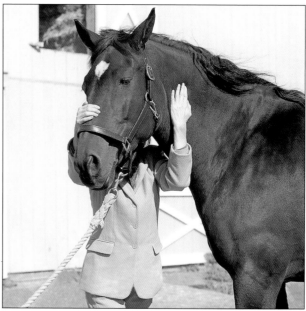

The Head

Working on the head and ears may have a profound effect on your horse. These techniques are therapeutic and extremely relaxing for both of you. You will have the opportunity to observe his facial expressions during work, something you were not able to do as you attended to the other areas of his body. You may wish to finish your session with all or some of these techniques, if he is comfortable being handled in this area.

Enjoy the varied expressions on Rocky's face as he communicates his feelings. Also keep in mind that we were indoors and for the first time in his long life, he was confronted with photography equipment (light reflectors and ladders) and flashes of light going off in his face. His cooperation and trust attest to his pleasure in this work.

THE EARS

There are acupuncture points in the ears that relate to the internal organs, and touching these points will have a general effect on the entire body, according to traditional Chinese medical theory. Also, the ears relate to the kidneys. I have read that, in the old days, Irish grooms massaged the ears of the horses in their care after hard work to help them recover their energy. There are seventeen muscles that are responsible for moving each ear. Working on the ears will have a positive and relaxing effect on the muscles of the poll area and down toward the eyes. Working the ears will help your horse through colic and it is beneficial to work on them while you are awaiting the vet. Concentrate on the tips of the ears for this.

If your horse is head shy, practice the holding position (as described below) without movement until he becomes accustomed to being touched here. When he is comfortable, begin your progression of techniques and remember that he is the boss. As you work, always accommodate your position and posture to his. Notice how I accomplish this in the following photos.

Ear rotations

Open your hand to the width of the base of his ears, with the index finger and thumb separated from the rest of your fingers. Place your hand at the base of his ear and mold it to the contours of his head. Take care not to pinch the ear. There should be hand contact through the entire palm area. The supporting hand is on his face if he accepts

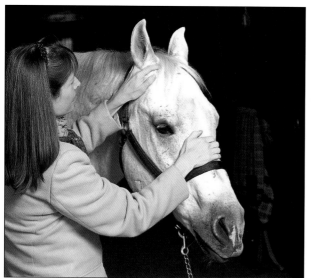
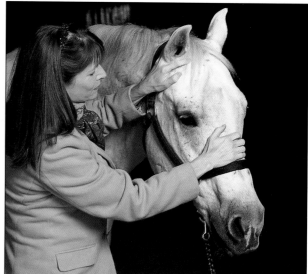

your touch here, otherwise hold him underneath his chin. Begin to rotate the hand that is holding the ear by pressing down gently and moving the skin at the base of the ear. Rotate in small circles in either or both directions several times. The Triple Heater and Gall Bladder Meridians pass through this area. Gradually stop rotating and without removing your hands from him, proceed to the next technique.

Walking the fingertips up the ear

This technique is done in whatever position he happens to be holding his ear. Using your thumbs on the inside and four fingers in contact with the outside of the ear, begin walking your fingers from the base to the top of the ear. This is done by moving your hands alternately. Do not reach too far inside his ears as it may tickle. Hold the point at the tip of his ear for several seconds before continuing to the next technique.

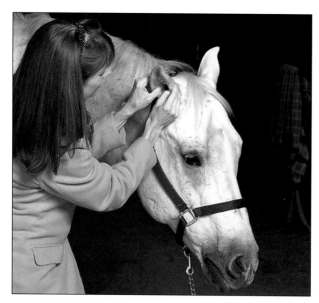
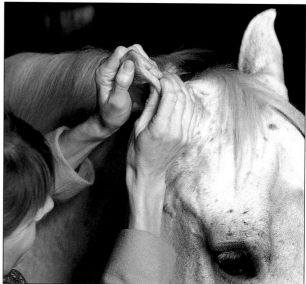

Ear traction

This is a variation of the previous technique, adding traction to the alternate fingertip-walking up the ear. Here *(left)*, I am leaning rearward, toward his tail, to stretch the tiny muscles in front of the ear. By alternately walking your left and right fingertips, you will be able to keep the ear stretched throughout the entire length to the tip. Do not pull the ear, just hold it back gently, then gradually release it without completely removing your hands.

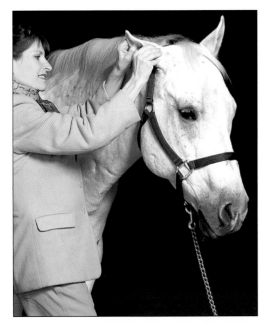

Now *(bottom left)*, I am drawing the ear outward, away from his head, toward my body, which is positioned facing his cheek. I am leaning back, away from him, having lowered my center to accommodate the increasingly relaxed body of my model. This release of the ear away from the head stretches the tiny muscles all around the base of his ear. Gradually release the traction without removing your hands from the ear and continue to the next technique.

Finish the ear traction with a forward stretch *(bottom right)*. This is a positive direction for ears, which is why I choose to end the ear stretches with this one. Walk your fingertips from the base toward the tip as you lean your body sideways, toward his nose. Notice how I have positioned my body as he lowers his head further down. Gently stretch the muscles behind the ear. Stop stretching gradually and repeat the ear rotation shown in the top two photos on page 130. Repeat the entire sequence on the other ear.

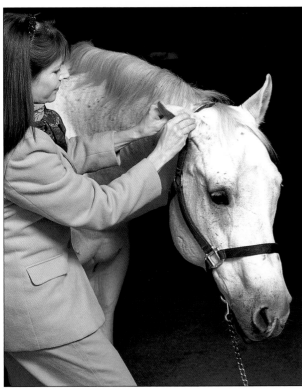

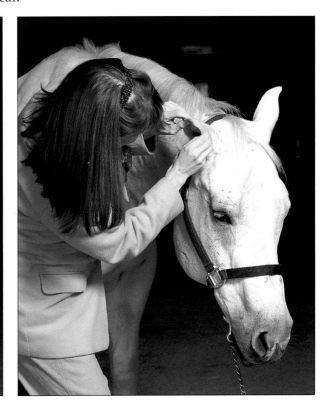

THE EYES

Make a smooth transition from the ear rotation on the second ear to the first eye technique, and keep contact with his body as you lower your hand to his eye. If you are working on his right eye, as shown, use your left hand for the upper portion and your right hand for the lower portion, making a smooth transition from one hand to the other. This is another relaxing area for you to attend to, as well as therapeutic. Also, keeping in frequent contact with his eye area aids drainage and circulation. You will find it easy to medicate him here if needed, since he will be accustomed to having your hands around his eyes. Be sure to clear any debris from his eyes before you begin.

Upper eye socket

I am working on the upper eye socket with my thumb. Place your supporting hand across his nose. Position your working hand so that the thumb rests against the underside of the bone above his eye. The little-finger side of your hand is resting against his forehead. Pressure is achieved by pressing your thumb toward your index finger; this motion will keep you from sliding into his eye. Keep your pressure going upward against the bone. Work from the inner corner of the eye along the upper eye socket in small increments, holding each point several seconds, to the outer corner of his eye.

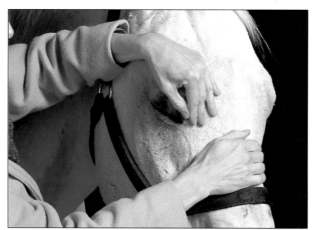
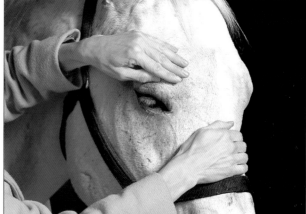
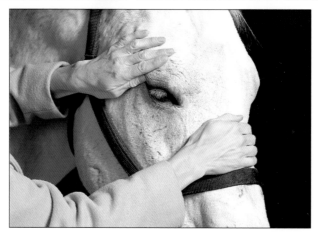

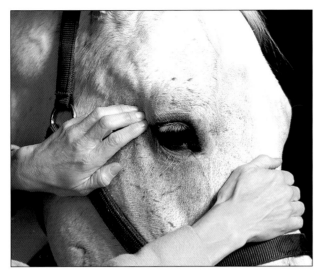 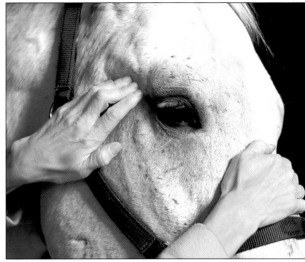

Outer corner of the eye

At the outer corner, align your four fingers against him and press in gradually and hold for several seconds. Then, without removing your fingertips or sliding on the hair, press gradually toward his ear, pulling the skin with you. This will help relax the muscles around the eye.

Lower eye socket

Change hands smoothly by slipping your current working hand under his head and placing it across his nose, it has now become your supporting hand. Use the fingertips of the other hand to work the lower eye socket moving from the outer corner toward the inner corner in small increments. Using your four fingertips, press downward onto the bone. The downward pressure will keep you from sliding toward his eyeball. Hold each point for a few seconds. Work toward the inner corner. Continue down the face toward the nose along the area of the tear duct.

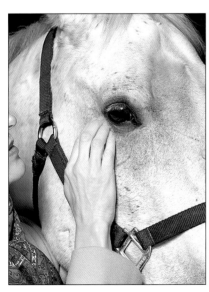 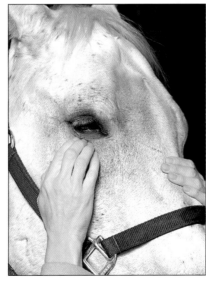 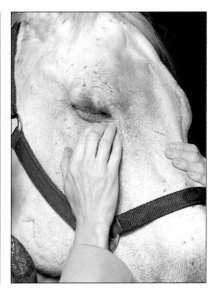

Working the tear duct

This technique is especially helpful for horses with allergies, nasal congestion and the tendency toward congested eyes.

Using the four fingertips, work down toward his nose from the inner corner of the eye. You may actually be able to feel the duct. To ensure that you touch it, position your fingertips parallel to the floor; you will cover a wider area this way. You may move your fingers in small circles, by moving the skin rather than sliding on top of the hair. Go slowly and patiently, and your efforts will be rewarded by a trickle of mucus from his nostril. Work in small increments, making several circles at each point. Your touch will be light and careful. Circle in either or both directions.

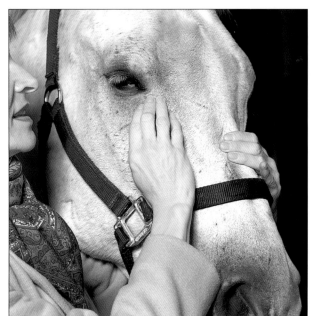
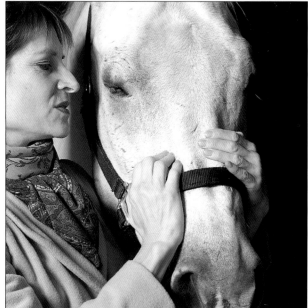
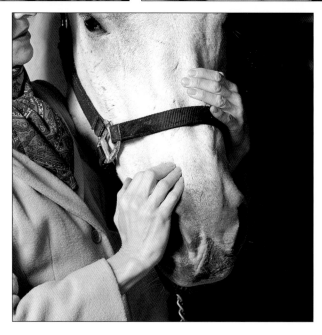

THE NOSTRILS

Working the nostrils will aid mucus drainage and help relax the muscles around his mouth.

Pulling the nostrils

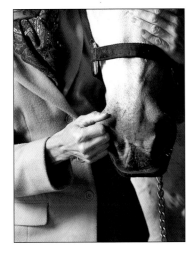

Making a smooth transition from the tear duct technique, you may now begin pulling the nostrils. Work each nostril after each tear duct. So, this sequence may be: one eye, its tear duct and nostril, then go to the other side.

Your supporting hand will go under his jaw and hold him across his nose. Take special care if he is wearing a halter not to press the strap into his skin, rather, hold him above or below the strap. Position yourself so that you are both facing the same direction.

First, softly grasp the nostril between your thumb and forefinger. Gradually squeeze the flesh around the outside of the rim of the nostril between these two fingers, simultaneously pulling it outward and holding it there for a few seconds. Release slowly and proceed to the next area, and work your way completely around, touching the entire tender circle of flesh. In these photos I am telling Rocky what a cute nose he has. He basks in compliments.

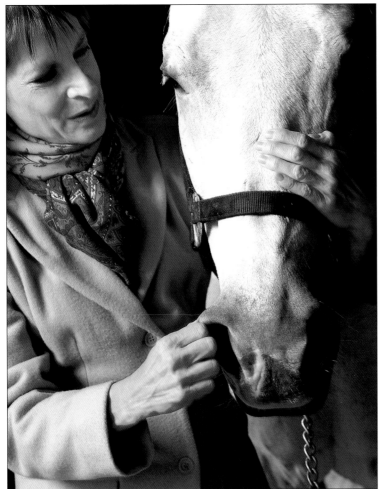

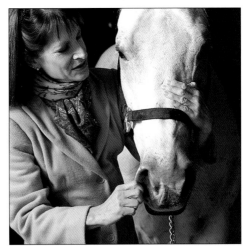

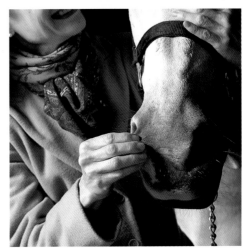

LOWER AND UPPER GUMS

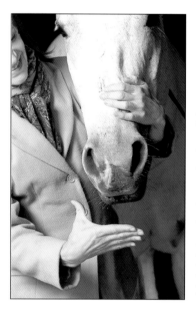

All horses have busy mouths; they are busy sorting through food, grooming and communicating. The upper lip is particularly active and expressive. Unhappy horses, or horses stressed by their environment, develop bad habits, many of which are centered around the mouth. Chewing their surroundings, and people, are typical expressions of their frustration. Working the mouth with the following techniques may relieve these habits, at least temporarily. These techniques are extremely relaxing and your horse may look particularly surprised the first time you do them. There are points on the lower and upper gums that you will be stimulating. This will help to keep your horse's teeth in healthy condition for years to come.

Sometimes when I am working on a particularly mouthy horse, who would like to chew on me as I work, I will do the mouth techniques first. This gives his mouth something to 'think' about, apart from working on me. Some horses want to groom me while I work on them. I do not encourage this as it distracts me and keeps them from concentrating on the sensations in their bodies. Also, as they begin to feel the effects of shiatsu they may become stimulated energetically and their ministrations to me may become painfully enthusiastic. If working on a stallion, you may generally wish to work on the head and mouth first.

Correct hand position

Open your hand and stretch the web between your thumb and forefinger. This stretched portion of your hand will contact the gums, well above the base of the upper teeth and below the base of the lower teeth. Depending upon the size of his mouth, you will adjust the shape of your hand to accommodate him. Your supporting hand is holding him across his face, from underneath. You will both be facing in the same direction.

Working the lower gums

I usually choose to work the lower jaw first, for if a horse has a tendency to raise his head, the slight downward pressure may prevent it.

Place the web of your hand on the top edge of his lower lip, molding it to the exact shape of the lip. Press downward, moving the lip away from the gums and position your hand on the gums as low as possible without forcing the movement. This will keep your hand away from the teeth.

Move your hand from side to side, molding it to the exact shape of his gums, covering the area below the teeth from your thumb, through the web of your hand to the index finger. Keep the contact complete. The pressure is fairly firm. Slide from side to side eight to ten times. If his mouth is dry, which may indicate nervousness, dip your hand into a bucket of water and try again. After working his lower jaw, remove your hand and give him a moment to 'digest' this technique. He will probably chew, lick, and even yawn.

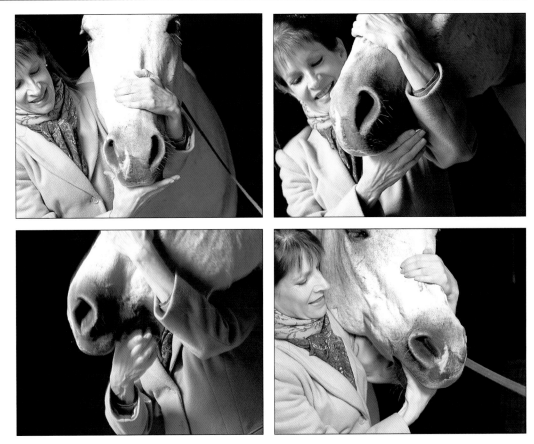

Working the upper gums Open your hand creating the web described on page 136. Place the web against his upper lip, molding it to the exact shape of the lip. Raise your hand, taking the lip upward with it, and tuck your hand under the lip against the gums well above the upper teeth. Slide your hand from side to side, molding it to the exact shape of his gums, eight to ten times. Remove your hand and give him a moment to appreciate the sensations.

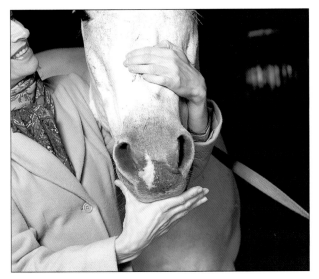

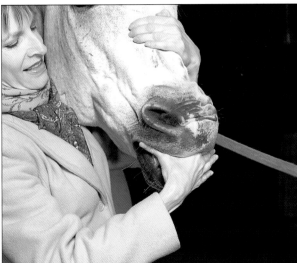

THE CHEEKS

Inside the cheeks

This is a powerful technique for releasing jaw, cheek and possibly neck tension. You may be surprised by the rough, damaged tissue inside some horses' cheeks. It will attest to the condition of their teeth. Releasing tension with this technique and work on the cheek from the outside, as follows, will change his facial expression and perhaps his entire attitude.

If your horse is still chewing and licking from the previous technique, wait until he has finished before starting work on the inside of the cheek, to avoid your fingers and his teeth getting to know each other too well. Keep your thumb against the inside of his cheek, well away from his teeth.

Initial contact

Place your supporting hand across his face and stand in front and slightly to the side of him. Slip the tip of your thumb into his mouth. Your four fingers are in contact with the outside of his face. Slide your thumb in, simultaneously lifting the skin until you feel it stretch and see some wrinkles near the corner of his mouth. Gently press your thumb toward the fingers on the outside of his face. Your supporting hand holds firmly but does not force his head down if he shows any objection to this technique.

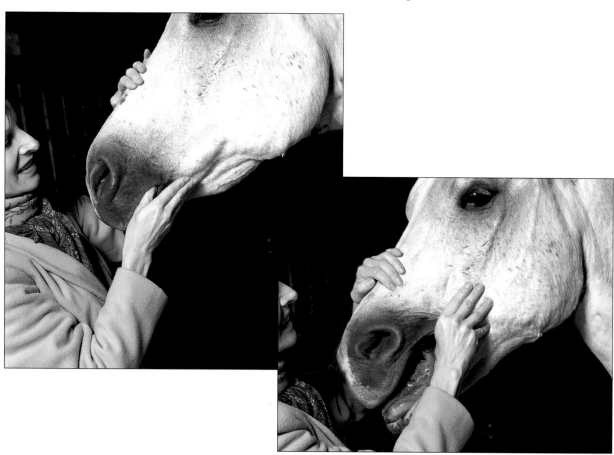

Stretching the cheek

Draw the skin downward as you press the flesh between your thumb and fingers. This is done by leaning your body rearward, so you will stretch gently and not pull forcefully. Accommodate his increasingly lowered head by dropping your center and lowering your body. Before you slide off his cheek, stop stretching, and press upward, repeating the technique three to five times. Before doing the other side, give him a moment to express himself.

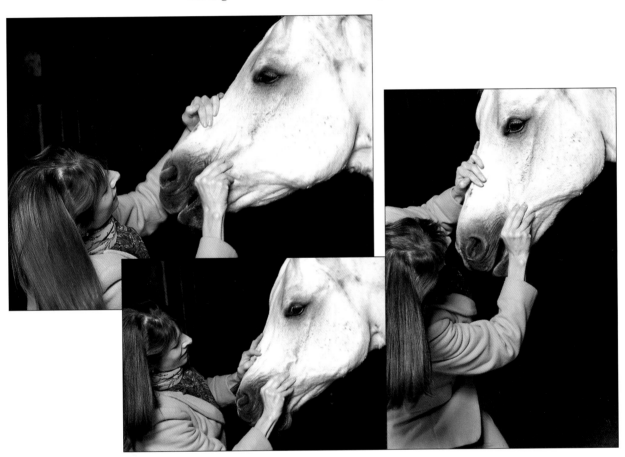

The cheek and jaw

To finish the work on the head, you will now work thoroughly on the cheek and jaw (from the outside). This is a large area and, to relax it thoroughly, you need to take some time. The muscles may be very tight and surprisingly sensitive (for both of you), so be patient and do not do more than he is comfortable with. If you, or someone you know, grinds their teeth, you will be familiar with the possibility of painful tension in the jaw and cheek muscles. Emotional problems as well as physical ones cause pain here. Improperly fitting bits, dental problems and inconsiderate riding are a few culprits. Jaw tension unrelieved will have negative consequences in other areas. Headaches are not uncommon as a result of jaw irritation; this will cause tension in the poll, upper neck, and onward. Imagine how frustrating it is for the horse if left unrelieved.

The jaw line

Stand facing his profile. Place your supporting hand softly across his face about halfway between his eyes and his nose. Use the little-finger side of your hand and place it just below his ear in the crease formed where his jaw meets his neck. You will have contact from the end of your little finger throughout its length, and the side of your hand. Then, lean in gradually at an angle vertical to the surface you are touching and slightly toward his nose. Work in small increments and hold each position for at least five seconds if possible.

In the photos below, I am working in the area where his jaw is close to his neck. Repeat the technique in this area a few times.

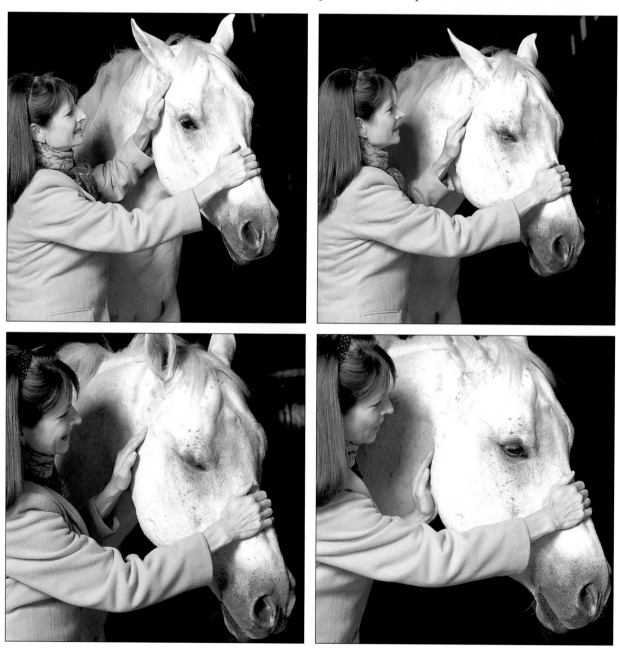

Here, where his jaw is free from his neck, I have changed my hand position. Use your thumb on the outside and four fingers, which are alongside each other, not spread out, on the underside of his cheekbone. Grasp the edge of the bone between your fingers, and squeeze gently. Use a flat thumb, not the tip. Your fingertips are also flattened, not pointed. This will be more comfortable for him and not cause him to feel poked.

Continue working toward his mouth as shown below by grasping the bone between your fingers. In the bottom photo I have changed the location of my supporting hand so you may easily see the position of my working hand.

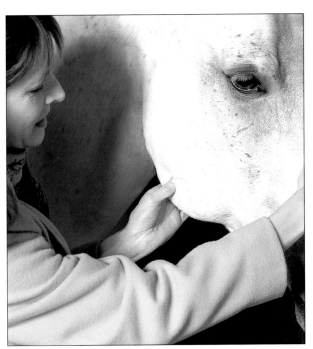
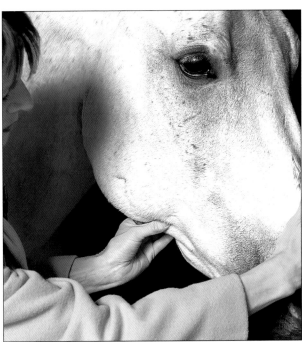

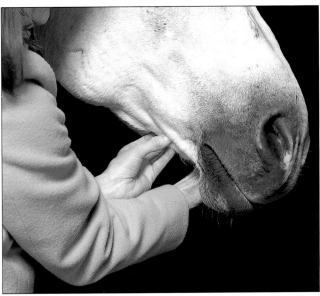

Muscles of the cheek

Place your palm heel on the lower edge of the cheek and press upward, without sliding, until you feel your hand filling with the muscle. Your supporting hand will go underneath his head to the opposite side and hold him as high on his head as possible, to support his head in a lowered position. Hold in each location for several seconds. Move your hand around to several locations where you are able to lift and move the muscles of his cheek. These locations are along the lower edge of his cheek. After a short time, you should feel the muscles get more pliant and yielding. He may be chewing and licking and lowering his head.

Work with your fingertips around the actual body of the cheek starting near his eyes and proceeding around until you have touched everywhere (possibly ten to fifteen locations). Use flat fingertips and align your fingers, rather than spreading them out. You may hold each location gently for several seconds or make circular motions, moving the skin under your fingertips, not sliding across the hair. You may wish to repeat the work you did inside his mouth, or proceed to the next technique.

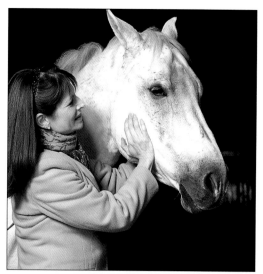
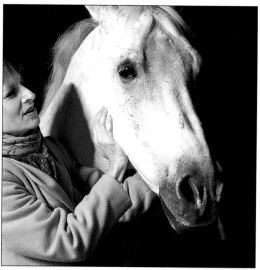
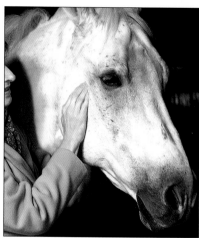
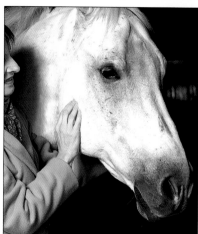
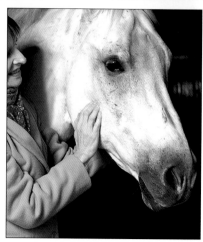

THE FOREHEAD

In the top two photos I am working down the center line of the forehead. Place your supporting hand on his poll. The weight of your relaxed hand is the only pressure on this area. Gather the fingertips of your working hand together and place them just below the forelock. Hold for five to ten seconds. Work in small increments toward a point just between his eyes and hold. Use steady holding pressure. The inward pressure is slow and steady, then hold, and release slowly and steadily. For example, count to five as you gradually increase pressure, hold while counting to five, and release to a count of five. Keep in contact with his forehead as you slide to the next location.

In the three bottom photos I am working with both thumbs simultaneously. This is a rare instance of no supporting hand being used. Place your thumbs next to each other, or one on top of the other, an inch or so below the forelock, then work outward along his brow in small increments. Remember to use your body to achieve pressure, even though the pressure may only be slight. On the first outward journey, the pressure is directly inward. You may then vary it, if you wish, to an outward stretching of these muscles. This is a wonderful finishing touch to the head and face work. His head may be so low that you are squatting to finish this technique. Slowly remove your hands and observe your now completely relaxed horse.

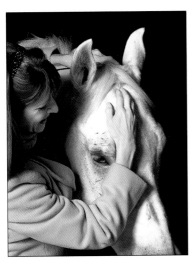
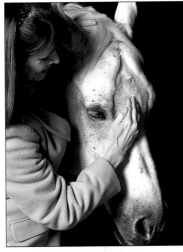
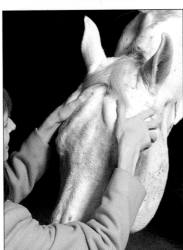
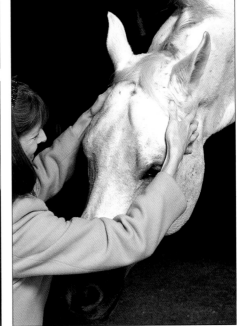

Finishing The Session

There are several scenarios that may follow the session. As much as we may want to stay near our horses after we finish the treatment, they do need their private time. I do not recommend that the horse be ridden immediately. He should have at least a fifteen minute period to enjoy the immediate effects of shiatsu. If the horse is an especially excitable type, and typically runs around the paddock when turned out, leave him in his stall for a time, then walk him in-hand for a few minutes before turning him out. The turnout time following treatment is especially valuable. The horse may then either calmly explore his environment, or stand meditatively. These reactions are desirable from a horse who likes to tear around his paddock. Some horses explore the new sensations in their bodies by moving from a deliberate walk to a long canter, complete with ebullient bucks. This is fine but should not go on for more than a few minutes. Keep him from using up the energy released by the session you have just finished. Many horses roll after shiatsu. Owners have told me that they had never seen their horses roll before, and many have told me that their horses had never rolled completely over before their first shiatsu session. Rolling is wonderful and gives them the opportunity to work out any kinks that you did not. You started the ball rolling with your session, and they are doing their own self-healing afterward. I love to stay with them as they express themselves after sessions, watching from a distance. Sometimes I do go into the paddock and run around with them a bit, because I feel so great after the session as well. Also, when I see how good they feel, it is hard not to dance around a little myself.

If the horse has a lameness problem, I suggest giving him at least one day of rest after the session, and wait until all signs of distress are gone before riding, or resuming any type of training.

Some horses' problems only show up when they are being ridden. In cases such as these, I may ask the owner to get on the horse after the fifteen minute rest period. The ride should be completely stress free and last just long enough to ascertain that movement has improved. You may see tremendous improvement following the first session but, of course, the saddle should have been checked to ensure a proper fit. Although I do not ride anymore, out of choice not necessity, and have only fairly limited experience of sitting on their backs, I do have an eye for balance and often can make very helpful suggestions to the rider while they are on their horse. I would never, however, contradict anything the trainer has said.

Of course, the rider's body is an important component in the balanced movement of the horse, so I usually check the rider's body during my first visit as well. This is done politely and unobtrusively. I encourage owners to observe my work on their horses during the actual session time. Most of them catch the relaxed vibration in the area and wish it were they who were receiving my treatment. Many begin to share their own complaints about their bodies with me. I usually invite them to sit on a trunk or hay bale after I finish with the horse and I work on their shoulders, arms, and sometimes necks, in a ten minute gift session. If I suspect they have a side to side imbalance in their bodies, or some other imbalance where I feel shiatsu would be appropriate, I suggest they have a full body session. I am often able to correlate their problem with their horse's imbalance. I may work with them for a few treatments as well as work on their horses. My business card says 'horse and rider shiatsu' because I know how important it is for both partners to feel comfortable in their precious bodies. Many owners take better care of their animals than they take care of themselves, and it may be difficult to convince them to have the session, so I talk to them about the harmony between partners being necessary for realizing the full potential of a good working and playing partnership.

One of the best situations is where I work on horse and rider the same day and they have a fun ride after I leave. I try to encourage an atmosphere of fun, and all of us together accomplishing something wonderful. I encourage people to play with their horses, with or without toys. Too many people get caught up in competition, and riding becomes a task with training and goals and no playfulness. This is so sad to me because I think we are here to enjoy ourselves and never to lose our childlike nature. Animals retain their innocence unless humans interfere. They can teach us so much about fun, exuberance and love. Shiatsu is a wonderful way to begin to listen.

Tall-horse Techniques

I always encourage harmonious movement between human and equine partners during shiatsu time. Sometimes it is difficult because of tremendous differences in size. My height is slightly above average (5 ft 6 in), so I manage to fit well with most horses. Some of my students are very short and can barely reach an average-to-tall horse's back. I encourage these people to have a specialty: ponies and small horses, although they valiantly try to work on horses who are huge next to them, and with good results too. If the student cannot reach the horse's back to work on it effectively, I remind them that working the back legs has an effect on the mid to low back, and working on the neck can have an effect on the entire back.

Some students are so tall that they have difficulty working on small horses or ponies. I always encourage creativity in taking my basic techniques and adapting them to the comfort of both partners. As long as you follow the principles of working from your center, supporting the horse and working with sensitivity and patience, you can adjust and compensate.

Here are some guidelines for working on a very tall horse. Neruda is 17.2 hh at the moment and still growing. He is sweet and agreeable as well as curious and talented. He and I will show you how to reach up and press down without force, but with effectiveness.

BEGINNING CONTACT   Establish your first contact with gentleness and love. Begin your session with all-over stroking as previously explained (*see* page 56).

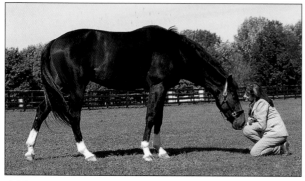

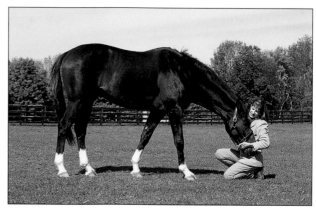

PALMING THE BACK

Use the supporting hand and working hand as usual. What is particularly important here is your body posture: you will reach up and place your hands on his back and it is important to lift your arms from the muscles underneath your arms and the muscles in your back (the latissimus dorsi) and not the muscles on top of your shoulders (upper trapezious). Keep your shoulders dropped even though your arms are raised. Make contact with your palms. To achieve pressure, drop your weight downward. Keep your knees soft rather than standing on your toes. The taller the horse, the more you have to drop your energy downward. You may need to stand closer to the taller horse to work. Keep your elbows soft throughout.

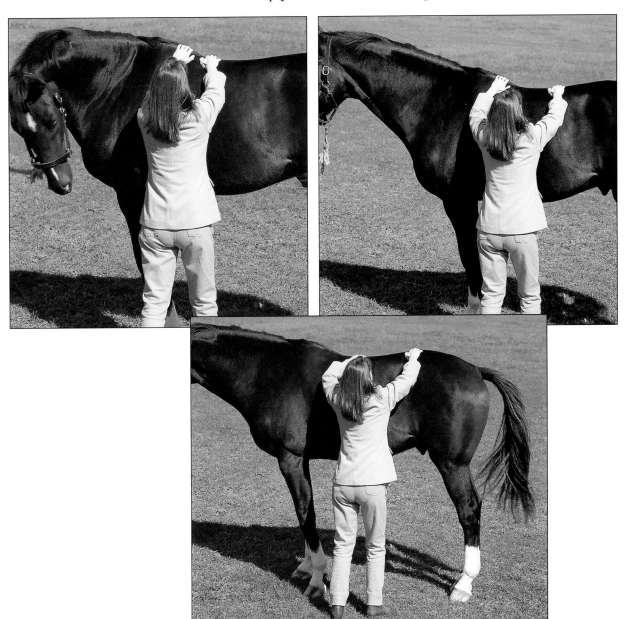

FINGERTIP PRESSURE ON THE BACK

Using the same principles as for palming, stand close to your horse and drop your weight downward. When working with the fingertips, keep the elbow of your working hand soft. Think of your elbow dropping downward to the ground. Once you have contact, begin dropping your weight straight through your center to the ground.

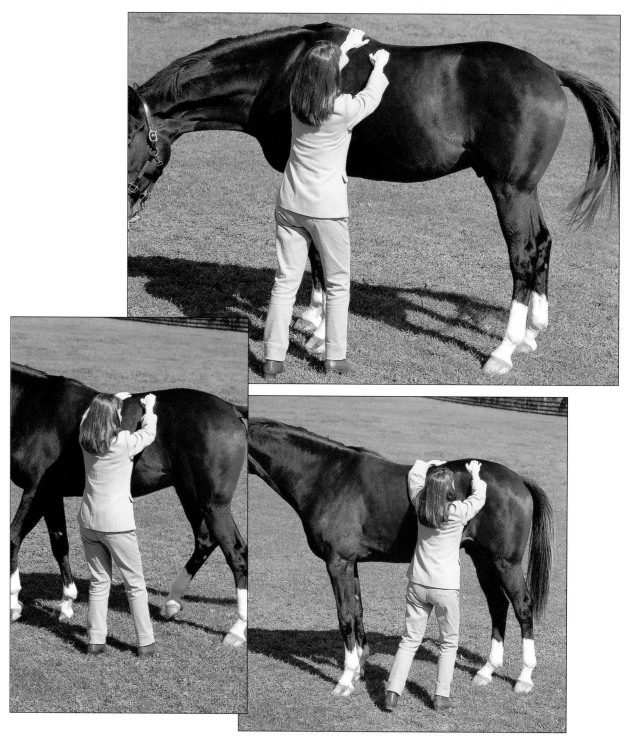

THE HINDQUARTERS

Since you will not be able to drape your supporting arm across to the other side of his body, hold near or on the Bladder Meridian. Work the hindquarters by reaching into the muscle without pushing him so that you do not force him to support himself too much with his far rear leg. Think of the contact rather than the push. Keep your working elbow soft. If it is too straight, you will be pushing him. Press in at different angles as well as vertically. If possible, grasp his back with your supporting hand, palm on one side and fingertips on the other side.

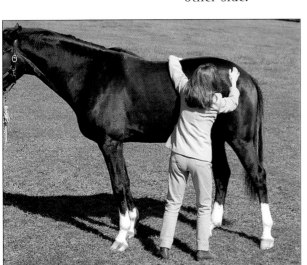
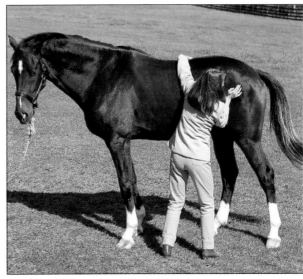

BLADDER MERIDIAN BEHIND THE LEG

Place your supporting hand as high on the croup as possible and point your fingertips toward his tail. Place the fingertips of your working hand in the meridian. Lean rearward toward his head to establish pressure. To keep tension out of your supporting arm, use the muscles under your arm and shoulder to reach up. Your shoulder muscles should be relaxed.

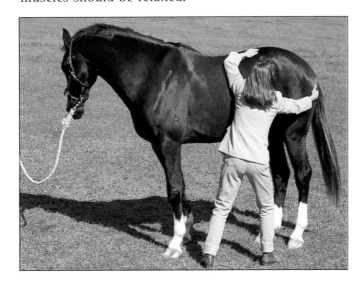

THE NECK STRETCH

Rudy is so tall it would be difficult to stretch his neck with his head in its normal position. It becomes easy to stretch him with his head lowered. Because he is young and curious, I have to make this into a game, with me in control of the rules of course.

The left-hand photo shows his neck beginning to curve but with his head tilted. This is not what I want. The other two photos show the corrected head position with him curling further and further around me. He seems to be giving me a hug. Notice that my supporting hand is across the top of his neck, as I have adapted to his lowered head position. Also notice that I am turning my body more each time, from my hips, as he bends around me.

One 'trick' is that the bigger they are, the smaller I want to make them feel. I want the really big ones, as well as the small ones, to feel cozy enough to curl up in my lap when I finish working on them. Sometimes huge horses are treated as if nothing could bother them but, often, these are the more sensitive creatures – gentle giants. I always try to look beyond the physical and into the heart.

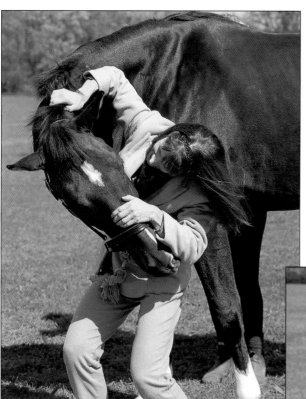

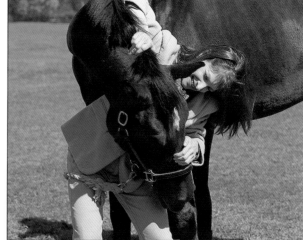

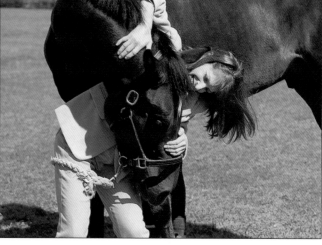

Ponies

When working with ponies we must use our body-weight in a different way. A lot of the techniques are done by leaning over, as well as squatting. Many of the back techniques are accomplished from the opposite side of the body. Also, the physical requirement of the pony's body is different from that of the horse, since most ponies are ridden by children or driven by adults. Still, they deserve to be comfortable in their bodies and happy in their hearts.

My model, Russell, is a very accomplished driving pony with a sweet disposition and clever mind.

In the following techniques, work using the principles of kyo and jitsu (*see* pages 246–9).

THE BACK AND HINDQUARTERS

Working the back with the supporting hand and working hand technique

Standing on one side of the pony facing his back, reach across to the opposite side and contact the Bladder Meridian, with your supporting hand on or near the withers, and work toward the hindquarters. By working from the far side, you can draw his body toward yours for his support and to accomplish your vertical pressure without pushing him away from you. The opposite foot to the working hand should be slightly behind you as usual. Your knees should be soft. Once your hands are in position on the Bladder Meridian, simply lean over from your center. Your shoulders must be relaxed. The pressure is actually directed a little toward your own body. Keeping contact with his body, walk to the other side and repeat.

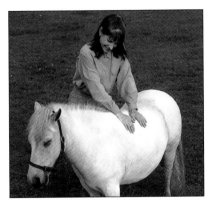
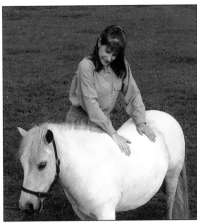
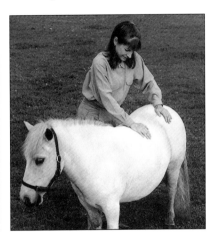

**Working the back
with both palms
simultaneously**

Place your palms on the Bladder Meridian, on both sides of his body. Step a bit away, and lean over, creating equal pressure in both palms. Your elbows should be bent as you lean into him. Work from the withers through the hindquarters, in small increments, staying aware of his reactions as you proceed.

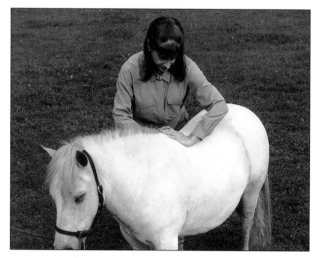
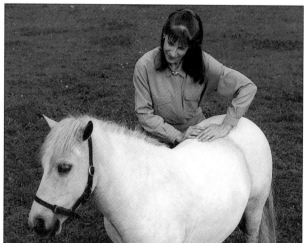

**Working the back with
the elbows**

Place your supporting palm on or near the withers and your working elbow nearby in the Bladder Meridian *(below left)*. Working from the opposite side, lean in, directing the pressure toward your own body. Work toward his hindquarters in this way, moving your supporting hand along to keep from getting too spread out. If you wish to use a stronger contact, you may bend the working arm slightly; this will make a more pointed surface of your elbow. If you lean in further, be sure to increase the pressure in your supporting hand. Never press with a pointed elbow initially; always go from a soft elbow to a pointed one and back to a soft one before proceeding to the next position.

Place both elbows in the Bladder Meridian. The elbows are soft. In this photo *(below right)*, my right elbow is the support. Keep your palms facing upward as you work along the back toward the point of hip.

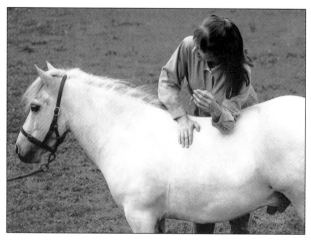
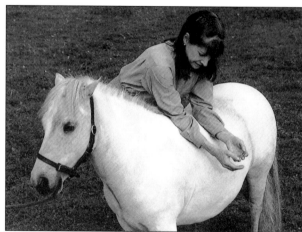

Stretching the Bladder Meridian

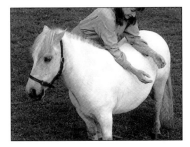

Hold these two points with equal pressure and, without sliding on the hair, stretch the area between them. This is accomplished by leaning in and separating your elbows. *(Left.)* Hold the stretch for several seconds, and slowly release.

Alternatively, cross your arms and place your palms between the withers and the point of hip *(below, left and right)*. Your palms are in the Bladder Meridian on the far side of his body. Without sliding, stretch the area between your palms by leaning over and dropping your body-weight over the area being stretched. You may place your left over your right or vice versa. Hold the stretch for several seconds, and slowly release.

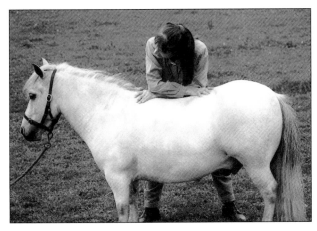

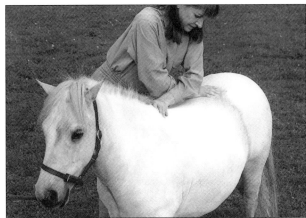

Working with one thumb

Start with your supporting hand at the withers as previously explained. Work on the Bladder Meridian with the thumb of your working hand *(below left)*. The thumb is soft, not pointed, and your fingers are lightly touching his body. Work both channels of the Bladder Meridian in this way.

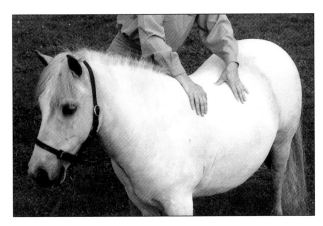

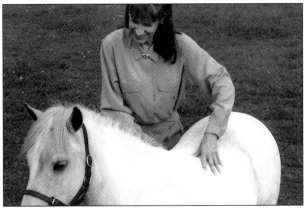

Working with both thumbs

Place both thumbs on the Bladder Meridian just behind the withers *(above right)*. Angle your body so you are facing slightly toward his head. Support your thumbs with your fingertips lightly resting on his body. Lean into your thumbs with gradual and equal pressure. Work in small increments (about the distance between vertebrae) and hold each point for several seconds, or until you feel energy moving under your thumbs.

Hindquarters

Support the hindquarters with your palm on the far side of the pony. Let your supporting palm mold to the curve of his body. Work the near side with your palm's heel. Your supporting hand is particularly important and will be equal in pressure to your working hand. This will keep you from pushing him away as you increase pressure with your working hand. Work all around his hindquarters, slowly and deeply.

Bladder Meridian in the hind leg

Place your supporting palm on the Bladder Meridian with fingers pointing toward the tail. Using the fingertips of the working hand, begin to work down the leg by leaning your body rearward to create the pressure in the meridian. The supporting hand is pushing toward the tail, to keep the pony's body stabilized. You are leaning over from the hips, with your knees bent and the opposite foot from your working hand behind you. Keep your body soft and try to keep your center in alignment with the points you are working on. As you get lower on the leg, your body is gradually sinking as well. When you reach the hock, smoothly lower your supporting hand, keeping it on the body and, from the inside of the leg, support with the fingertips of the hand just above the hock. Be sure the fingertips of the supporting hand are in the meridian. The supporting hand's fingertips are holding but not pulling. Continue toward the last point at the hoof.

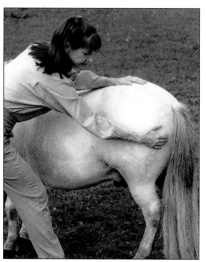
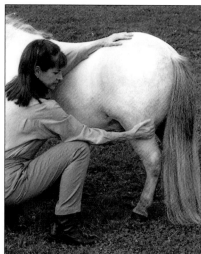
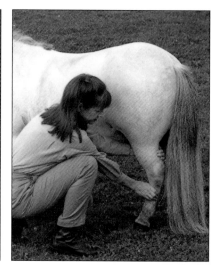

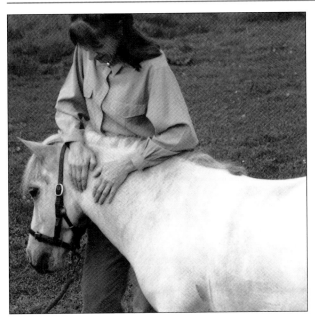
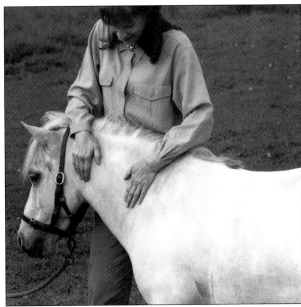

THE NECK

Neck meridians

Work from the opposite side to the treatment area and use your body for support. The supporting hand, near the head, holds the pony's head gently and securely against your body. Your working hand, using the palm and/or fingertips, can work on the neck meridians. Do both sides to determine if one is more sensitive than the other. *(Above left and right.)*

Lengthening neck stretch

Supporting his head against your body, encourage him to lower his head until his neck is resting on or near your upper thigh. Bend your leg and lean away, holding firmly at the neck near the shoulder and stretching his neck forward. This is done very gradually, and released very gradually. Do not remove your hands as you proceed to the next technique. You may incorporate a slight side stretch by turning your body. *(Below left and right.)*

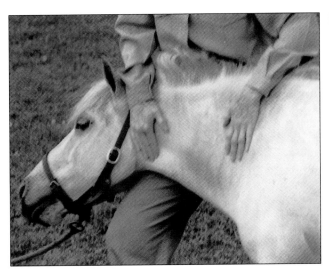
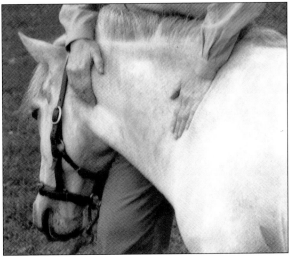

Alternative lengthening neck stretch

This alternative stretch is done with the practitioner squatting next to the neck. Hold the pony under the chin and at the top of the neck, just a bit behind the poll. Lean your body sideways until you feel the neck begin to stretch and lengthen. Hold here for several seconds and slowly release.

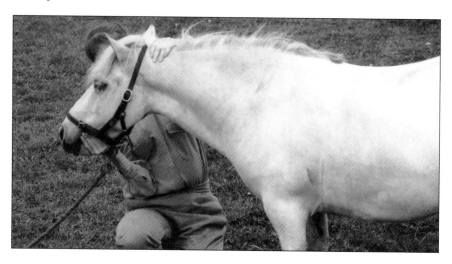

Incremental neck exercise

Always begin on the pony's less sensitive side if he has one. Squat and support his head from underneath. Place your working hand on the center line of the neck. Hold the neutral position, then turn the head slightly toward you. Release it back to the neutral position, move your hand along an inch or two, and move the head again. This is not a stretch, rather, small movements to define the movement of each neck vertebra. Work on both sides.

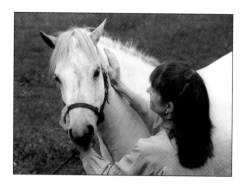

Neck side stretch

Still squatting alongside the pony, place your working hand on the center line of the neck and closer to the horse's head than to his withers. As your hand works toward the shoulder in increments of two to three inches, bend his head around smoothly to stretch the neck. Try to make a wide arc so as not to compress one side as you stretch the other. Keep his head from twisting and hold at the first point of resistance. Then, perhaps, release a bit, and then stretch a little more. Release to a neutral position with the support of both hands. Stretch both sides beginning with his less-stiff side.

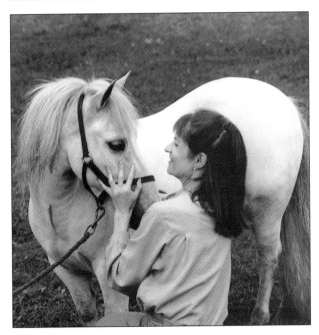
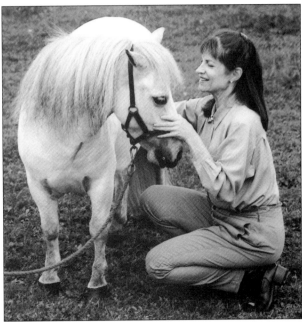

Alternative neck side stretch

First, place your hip against his neck in front of his shoulder. Hold the far side of his neck with your palm and forearm. Hold him across his nose, taking care not to press his noseband into his face. Using your body as a fulcrum, wrap his neck around you without pulling. Hold him here and, if he feels safe and comfortable, turn your body, taking his head with you and curving his neck around your hip. Hold him here for several seconds, or as long as he wishes, and slowly release, with your hands still on him, and then repeat on the other side.

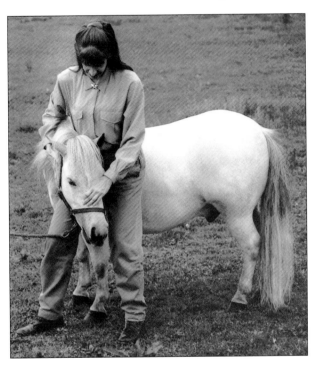
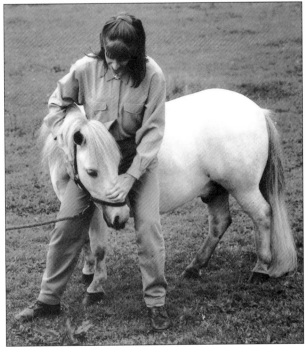

THE FRONT LEGS

Leg rotation position

Squat to the outside of the pony's leg facing his hindquarters and lift his foot off the ground until the lower leg is parallel to the ground. Rotate it by moving your body in a circular motion and taking the leg with you. The rotation is done in either or both directions, from three to ten times. You may begin with very small rotations, and increase the diameter gradually. Be sure the pony keeps his balance. You may proceed to any of the foreleg techniques, as practiced on horses, by adjusting your body position.

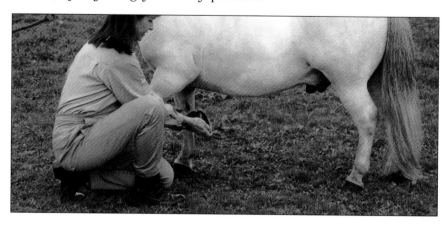

Leg stretch

Making a smooth transition from the rotation position, straighten the pony's leg and hold with one hand behind the knee and the other hand behind the pastern. Keeping his foot fairly low to the ground, drop your body-weight into your hips and lean rearward, gradually stretching his leg. In this position, your noses will be at about the same level, so be prepared for sniffs, snuggles, and snot!

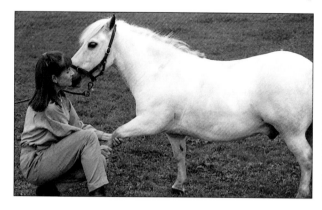 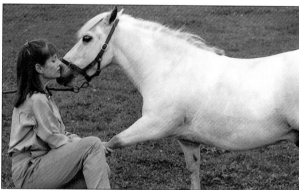

THE SHOULDERS

Shoulder technique suggestions

Either face in the same direction as your pony or toward the rear of the pony and work the shoulder while holding at the withers with your supporting hand, or place the supporting hand on the opposite side of the neck. Work the meridians of the shoulder with the palm and fingertips or simply press generally into several areas of the shoulder muscles. Your body should be bent at the waist, knees slightly bent, and back straight. *(Opposite, top three photos.)*

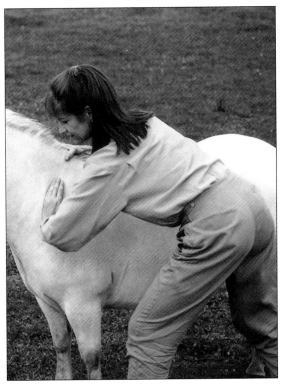
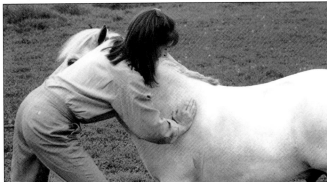
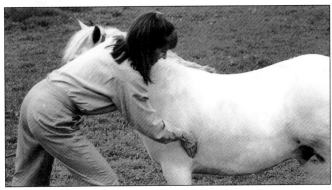

THE BACK LEGS

Rotation of the back leg

From a squatting position, lift the pony's leg and hold it under the fetlock joint with the inside hand and under the hoof with the outside hand (below left). Keep the foot low to the ground and rotate the leg by moving your body in a circular motion. This may be difficult in your squatting position, so concentrate on moving from your center. Keep the leg lifted and continue to the leg stretch.

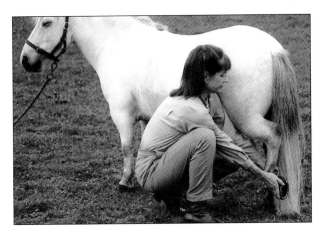
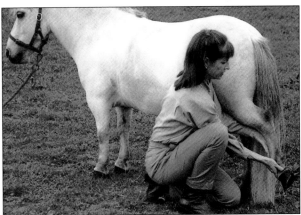

The back leg stretch

Adjust your hand positions so that each hand is a bit higher on his leg. Shift your weight forward to stretch the leg directly rearward (above right). Your inside knee may be touching the ground at this point. Hold in this position for several seconds and keep the leg lifted for the next technique.

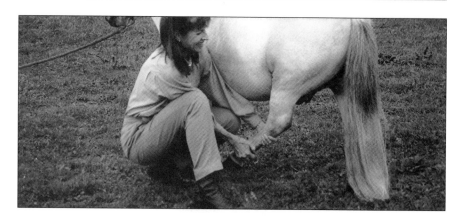

Back leg forward stretch

Still squatting, begin to lean your weight into your hips as you change your hand position to wrap around the back of his leg. Your hands should be separated for maximum support. Take his rear leg directly toward his front leg, keeping the hoof low to the ground. Without placing the foot down, shift your weight by leaning forward and repeat the rearward stretch. Repeat this sequence of rotation and stretches on the other leg.

You may practice any of the other leg techniques by adjusting your body position to lower your center of gravity to accommodate his body dimensions.

THE HEAD

Lower your body and work the eyes as explained on pages 132–4.

The eyes

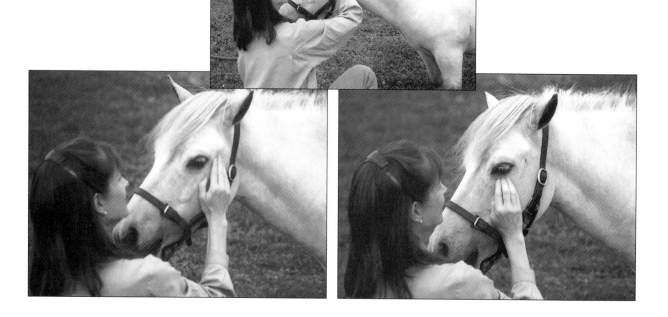

The ears   Work the ears as explained on pages 129–31.

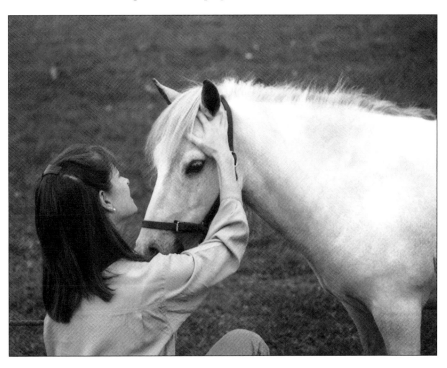

The mouth   Work the mouth as explained on pages 136–8.

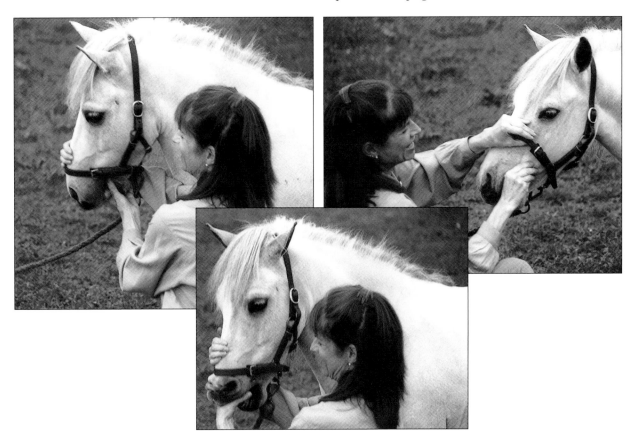

Releasing tension at the poll

Bend from the waist, keeping your back straight, with your knees slightly bent. Hold your pony at the poll, with your thumb on one side and four fingers on the other. The four fingers are aligned, with their sides touching. The other hand holds across his nose. Rock his head from side to side in small movements as you apply gentle and steady pressure at the poll. Gradually stop rocking.

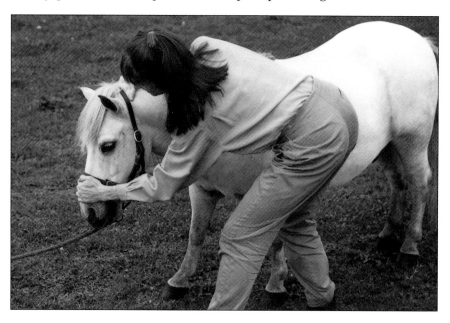

THE TAIL

See the guidelines for tail work for horses on pages 109–115 while adapting your body position to work on the pony's tail. Lower your-self so you can lean rearward, drawing the tail back on the same line on which it comes out of the body. Keep your back straight and have your hands separated.

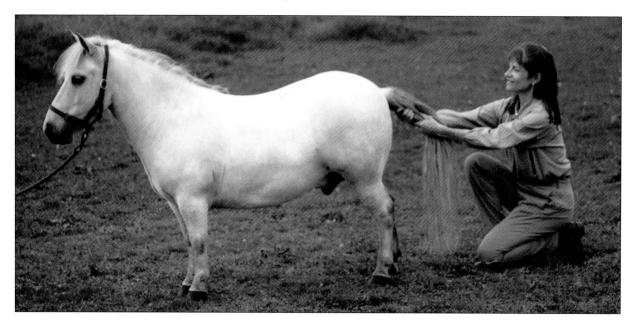

Children and Shiatsu

I always encourage children and teenagers to work on their horses. This gives a youngster and their horse a good way to communicate and understand each other, whether the relationship is new or has been established over time. Children are very good practitioners because their bodies have not developed the tension a lot of adults have, and their attitudes are joyous with the spirit of fun. They also have no preconceived ideas or expectations. Shiatsu is fun!

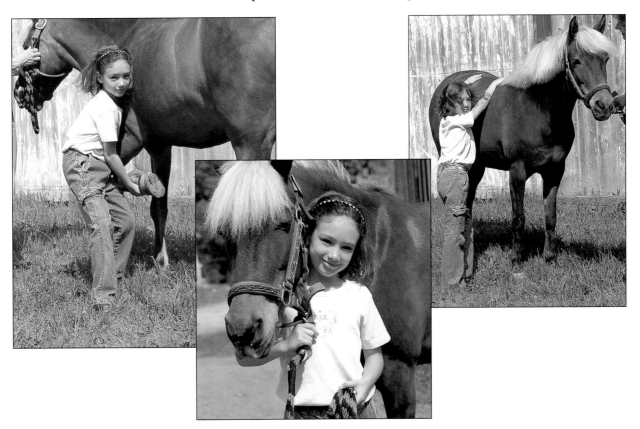

Jacqui Lloyd works on her pony Cinnamon. By correct body placement, the pony's leg did not seem too heavy. Jacqui is still too small to do stretches, but she can work on her pony's back, tail, face, and do some rotations. This pony takes very good care of her little girl, who loves her very much.

Jacqui's older sister, Emily, works on her new horse Sylvester (having outgrown Cinnamon). Emily took my Level 1 course with her mother Debbie (Rocky the head model's mommy) shortly after getting Sylvester. They bonded during the course and Emily's work on his face and in his mouth elicited multiple yawns.

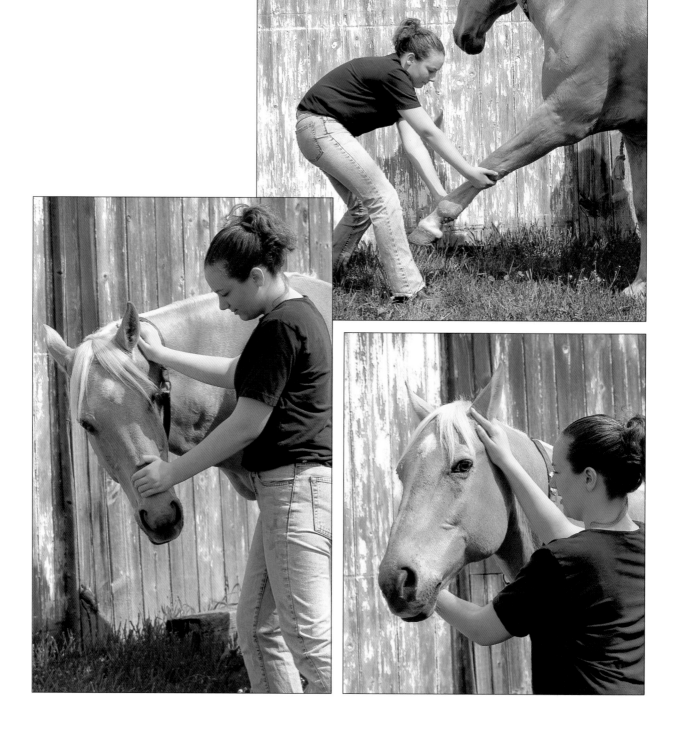

Part IV

THE MERIDIANS:
CHARACTERISTICS AND CHARTS

LUNG AND LARGE INTESTINE MERIDIANS (Lu AND LI)
Lung Meridian (yin)

Function	Governs the intake of life energy through the air, and governs resistance to external intrusions, such as airborne pathogens, dust and allergens etc., and has, therefore, an important function in immunity. It also relates to the skin, the largest organ of elimination. The Lung Meridian also governs elimination of gases through exhalation. *Wei chi*, the protective energetic field produced by the lungs, regulates energy throughout the body through respiration.

Optimal functioning condition

Physical characteristics	Soft subtle skin that heals well with little scarring, healthy coat quality, lean body type with lovely and elegant features, and healthy sweat glands. Quick recovery from illness.
Emotional characteristics	These horses interact well in their environment, approach situations with intelligence, are safe (perhaps bombproof) and quiet. They adapt well to new situations and enjoy the challenge. It is best to handle these horses patiently with clear instructions and respect. They should be given a variety of tasks to avoid the boredom of routine. They are social and interact well with their people as well as others in their herd.

Kyo manifestation

Physical characteristics	There may be difficulty in breathing and shortness of breath, a susceptibility to colds, fatigue from work, running eyes and nose, weight gain due to elimination problems, shoulder pain, chronic cough, thin liquid running from the nose, weak shoulders and narrow chest.
Emotional characteristics	These horses are overanxious and sensitive, avoid contact with other horses and people, hold old emotions such as grief memories, loss, and may show characteristic aloofness. In extreme cases there may be complete emotional shutdown. These horses may be withdrawn.

Jitsu manifestation

Physical characteristics	Prone to colds where there is stagnation, thick nasal discharge, excessive coughing, constipation, bronchial problems, tight chest muscles, shoulder pain, poor coat quality, difficulty in skin healing, inefficient and inconsistent sweating, fluid accumulation, urination problems, edema, and difficulty in bouncing back after illness. Skin irritations such as flaking, and allergic reactions to many things. Also, abnormal hair growth, and shoulder problems.
Emotional characteristics	These horses show: an inability to release tension when upset over small details, emotionally induced coughing, aggressive behavior toward other horses and people, difficulty in taking deep breaths to release tension. These horses may be withdrawn emotionally and emanate a deep emotional sadness and grief over unresolved long past events.

Large Intestine Meridian (yang)

Function

Assists the function of the Lung Meridian. Moves turbid parts of food and fluid as it absorbs fluid from this waste material. Controls the formation and elimination of feces. Eliminates stagnation of energy.

Optimal functioning condition

Physical characteristics

Easy recovery from physical disturbances, such as injuries which involve inactivity, change in environment, travel. Clear breathing passages.

Emotional characteristics

Mature, emotionally stable horses who easily forgive occasional awkward efforts of handlers.

Kyo manifestation

Physical characteristics

Dry or congested nasal passages, or clear mucus running from the nose, prone to diarrhea resulting from change in diet, travel or ingestion of coarse food, pus or mucus formation around the eyes and nose, very susceptible to skin inflammation, and poor abdominal circulation. Poor resistance to colds and allergies.

Emotional characteristics

These horses can develop diarrhea for emotional rather than physical reasons, can become overly dependant upon a handler and have emotional swings due to elimination disturbance and ensuing headaches.

Jitsu manifestation

Physical characteristics

Nasal congestion, bronchial disturbances, chronic constipation problems, headaches, itchy or inflamed skin, cough, anal irritation.

Emotional characteristics

These horses can be inconsistent performers, have unpredictable mood swings and seemingly unexplainable grumpy behavior.

SPLEEN AND STOMACH MERIDIANS (Sp AND St)
Spleen Meridian (yin)

Function	Governs digestion, including all digestive juices, reproductive hormones and secretions from the small intestine. Internal branches go to the stomach, spleen, pancreas, heart, and mouth. Assists immune system by detecting foreign bodies in the blood. The spleen is a storehouse for red blood cells which supply extra oxygen to the muscles, and extracts nutrients from food to create blood.

Optimal functioning condition

Physical characteristics	Good energy level and appetite, healthy immune system, 'easy keepers' (good doers), good teeth, good digestion, good dense muscle tone.
Emotional characteristics	These horses are not overly bothered by external stresses, are 'solid citizen' types, can eat under any condition with good digestion and elimination and are reliable and steady, although they function best in their own environment.

Kyo manifestation

Physical characteristics	Dry mouth, sticky saliva, thirst, drink a lot with food, poor digestion, backache, pale gums, anemia, weak immune system, weak thin body, dental problems, chronic diarrhea, dull coat with skin problems such as rain scald (rain rot), weak muscles which respond slowly to conditioning programs, sway backs due to being overweight.
Emotional characteristics	These horses have poor memories, are restless and anxious, shy and nervous, lack concentration, and are prone to diarrhea due to emotional upset.

Jitsu manifestation

Physical characteristics	Gastric hyperactivity, stomach inflammations, being overweight and overeating, stiff and tight muscles, tightness in the abdomen and navel area, craving sweet foods, dental problems, chronic and acute colic, diarrhea, fluid retention, windpuffs (windgalls) in hind legs, hay belly.
Emotional characteristics	These horses suffer from mental unrest, overthinking and worrying, shyness to the point of isolation from others, are overly cautious, and crave sweet foods.

Stomach Meridian (yang)

Function | Related to the function of the stomach and the digestive tubes. In females it relates to the function of reproduction, including lactation, ovary function and estrus. Also relates to appetite mechanism.

Optimal functioning condition

Physical characteristics | Good strong metabolism characterized by a broad body and rounded abdomen. Good appetite and digestion. Strong, solid features overall.

Emotional characteristics | These horses have a good appetite for life, including associations with people and other animals. They require stability of routine. They are extremely loyal and patient, and mentally well grounded (therefore safe mounts for even inexperienced riders), with good endurance.

Kyo manifestation

Physical characteristics | Bad breath, bloated stomach, sinus problems, stiffness and tiredness without reason, lack of sufficient gut sounds, unpleasant gas smells, poor appetite or eating without appetite, diarrhea, or constipation, easy weight gain, low energy and lethargic behavior. In mares, unregulated estrus and difficulty in conceiving.

Emotional characteristics | These horses are preoccupied and moody, have a poor appetite or are uninterested in food, crave sweet foods, overreact for too long to a change in environment, have their heads in the clouds without their feet being firmly on the ground, are lethargic and sluggish, depressed, worriers who easily lose weight.

Jitsu manifestation

Physical characteristics | Heaviness in the stomach, easy weight gain, jaw tension and grinding of teeth, and digestion problems due to misaligned jaw joint, frequent colic, tight muscles, stifle problems. Congestion in female reproductive system.

Emotional characteristics | These horses think too much and are therefore neurotic, rushing around needlessly, are nippy because of craving for food, always looking for food, and become aggressive if not fed first or on time. Mares show overprotective behavior and difficulty during weaning process and, also, may have a tendency to 'steal' other mares' foals.

HEART AND SMALL INTESTINE MERIDIANS (Ht AND SI)
Heart Meridian (yin)

Function	Governs emotions and blood circulation. Assists in adapting external stimuli to the body's internal environment via the brain and five senses.

Optimal functioning condition

Physical characteristics	Efficient blood circulation which nourishes tissues and flushes away waste products, healthy gums and tongue.
Emotional characteristics	These horses are fiery at appropriate times, such as competitive events, and friendly, calm and gentle afterward. They adapt well to outside stresses.

Kyo manifestation

Physical characteristics	Easily fatigued, poor circulation, constitutional weakness, abnormal pulse, exercise intolerance.
Emotional characteristics	These horses are oversensitive, unresponsive socially, depressive, joyless and stoic, and have a lack of determination and a sluggish mind.

Jitsu manifestation

Physical characteristics	Poor circulation to the extremities, digestive problems, palpitations and irregular heartbeat, and abnormal tongue color.
Emotional characteristics	These horses are chronically tense, fatigued, hyperactive mentally, restless, panic easily, and are overly affectionate with annoying habits such as licking, cribbing, and not calming down after emotional highs.

Small Intestine Meridian (yang)

Function

Small Intestine governs the entire body. It assimilates nutrients from food, conducting fluid waste to the kidneys and solid waste to the large intestine. Small Intestine assists the heart in communication from within and without the body by the purification and transportation of fluids and substances that enter the blood. It registers mental anxiety and nervous shock first, to protect the entire body.

Optimal functioning condition
Physical characteristics

Good digestion and circulation.

Emotional characteristics

These horses are joyful and courageous, charming and enthusiastic, exhibit friendly behavior and will be playful with a sense of humor. The life spark is always alight.

Kyo manifestation
Physical characteristics

Erratic elimination, irregular body temperature, anemia, blood stagnation, female reproductive problems, shoulder pain and headaches.

Emotional characteristics

These horses are cold with little or no emotional spark, overly cautious and timid and easily depressed. They are unable to discern relevant details of the job at hand, and therefore easily distracted by outside influences, and have poor concentration.

Jitsu manifestation
Physical characteristics

Poor circulation in the extremities, shoulder stiffness, headaches, stiffness of the cervical vertebrae, and reproductive problems in mares.

Emotional characteristics

These horses are constantly all fired up, lose their cool easily and have trouble calming down again. Mental activity keeps them from concentrating on their work. They may anticipate their riders' needs rather than listening to cues.

KIDNEY AND BLADDER MERIDIANS (K AND BI)
Kidney Meridian (yin)

Function	Filters pure fluid from turbid fluid to produce urine, related to inherited energy, governs all body fluids, including tears, saliva, mucus, urine, sweat, cerebrospinal fluid, plasma, and semen. Controls spirit and energy. Detoxifies and purifies blood.

Optimal functioning condition

Physical characteristics	Energetic, without suddenly burning out, efficient urination, without emotional holding, and soft but strong back muscles.
Emotional characteristics	These horse are ambitious, learn easily with concentration, are well adjusted to change and they regulate energy flow with an internal intelligence.

Kyo manifestation

Physical characteristics	Cold backed, frequent urination, difficulty in regaining energy after work, therefore longer recovery time, cracked hooves and malfunctioning hormone production. Stiffness from behind the saddle area to the quarters, splitting hooves, and a predisposition to bone fractures.
Emotional characteristics	These horses are fearful and anxious, constantly in need of reassurance, have a complaining body language, a lack of determination and no sense of adventure.

Jitsu manifestation	**Kidney Meridian is rarely jitsu and, if it is, it is often jitsu hiding kyo.**
Physical characteristics	Stiffness in back, frequent urination with densely colored urine, bladder problems, poor circulation, arthritic with bony overgrowth, easily dislocated low back.
Emotional characteristics	These horses are nervous and anxious, restless, spook easily, have a lack of determination, and keep going beyond the point of exhaustion with consequent burnout physically and emotionally.

Bladder Meridian (yang)

Function

Regulates the flow of energy in all the meridians, as well as assisting the actual urinary function of receiving and excreting urine. It is related to the midbrain, which cooperates with the pituitary gland and kidney hormone system. It is related to the autonomic nervous system.

Optimal functioning condition
Physical characteristics

Good stamina and sexual energy.

Emotional characteristics

These horses are confident and mature, patient and steady, resilient and are survivors. They can go with the flow in many situations and can be fearless and cautious simultaneously.

Kyo manifestation
Physical characteristics

Dislocations of the neck at the poll and spinal dislocations happen easily and are difficult to set right. Cold backed. Hock and stifle joint problems.

Emotional characteristics

These horses have a lack of patience, are fearful of new situations, do not handle change well, have a lack of desire to learn new things, are anxious and timid, even depressed, and emotional tension results in body tension.

Jitsu manifestation
Physical characteristics

Tightness in the back of the leg, frequent urination, neck tightness and tired eyes. Back pain and tension, with a tendency toward tying up (azoturia), and the need for a long warm-up time.

Emotional characteristics

These horses are oversensitive, fuss over trivialities, are mentally inflexible and stubborn, overly aggressive at times and forge through thoughtlessly.

LIVER AND GALL BLADDER MERIDIANS (Li AND GB)
Liver Meridian (yin)

Function	Stores blood and releases nutrients and energy for physical activity, purifies blood of waste products, stores and releases blood, governs flow of energy, relates to the muscles and connective tissues, hooves, eyes, reproductive organs and resistance to disease.

Optimal functioning condition

Physical characteristics	Muscles recover quickly from activity, bright eyes and healthy hooves, strong joints, good sexual energy (especially in males).
Emotional characteristics	These horses are even tempered, hard workers with good concentration, determined and consistent and have a good appetite.

Kyo manifestation

Physical characteristics	Easily strained tendons, weak joints and muscles, tendency to stumble because of overall lack of energy and eye problems, easily poisoned by any toxic substances because of inability to detoxify quickly, impotence with lack of sexual energy.
Emotional characteristics	These horses are easily upset, nervous, have a lack of determination, and a tendency toward tiredness, depression and mood swings in mares relating to their heat cycle.

Jitsu manifestation

Physical characteristics	Inflammation of the female or male reproductive organs, flatulence, muscle spasms, tying up (azoturia), headaches, eye problems, cracked dry hooves, lack of sexual energy, weak joints and muscles, exhaustion.
Emotional characteristics	These horses are stubborn, work tirelessly until exhausted, are prone to angry displays with quick resolution, show aggressive behavior and must be in consistent work to overcome inconsistent behavior, sexual aggression, and have habits such as weaving, pacing (box walking), cribbing and biting.

Gall Bladder Meridian (yang)

Function	Governs secretions such as bile, saliva, gastric acid, insulin and intestinal hormones, and helps distribute nutrients. Although horses do not have gall bladders, they do possess a system that governs the flow of bile to the liver.

Optimal functioning condition

Physical characteristics	Good muscle tone, gradual expenditure of muscular energy without sudden fatigue, good digestion, excels at dressage.
Emotional characteristics	These horses are mentally flexible and able to make sensible decisions, therefore may be less prone to becoming injured, and may be a safe mount because of this ability.

Kyo manifestation

Physical characteristics	Tired muscles, poor digestion, with a tendency toward diarrhea or constipation, eye problems such as poor sight, mucus formation, gastric hyperacidity and poor distribution of nutrients in spite of a good diet, easily dislocated joints because of a lack of healthy elasticity of the ligaments and tendons, and hind end lameness.
Emotional characteristics	These horses are hypersensitive, timid, have a lack of determination, lack of spirit, are indecisive, followers rather than leaders, and are easily taken advantage of by people and other horses.

Jitsu manifestation

Physical characteristics	Prone to lameness resulting from stiffness in muscles, exhaustion because of energy burnout, explosive energy bursts due to lack of regulation in the meridian system, headaches, neck problems, eye problems, bloated stomach, mucus problems, coughing and poor appetite.
Emotional characteristics	These horses are easily upset with a physical reaction that may be explosive, irritable, angry, possibly to the point of aggression, stubborn, and show too much attention to small details.

HEART CONSTRICTOR AND TRIPLE HEATER MERIDIANS (HC AND TH)
Heart Constrictor Meridian (yin)

Function	Supports the function of the Heart Meridian and governs circulation throughout the body via the system of veins and arteries. Related to the heart sac and cardiac artery, and controls total nutrition. Acts as a buffer for the Heart Meridian both physically and emotionally.

Optimal functioning condition

Physical characteristics	Good circulation with network of veins appearing on the body during work, and the ability to cool down easily, also, quick recovery from high fever and performance stress.
Emotional characteristics	These horses recover quickly from emotional agitation and anxiety, such as adjusting to a new owner, or being moved to a new environment and leaving old friends.

Kyo manifestation

Physical characteristics	Malfunctioning of the heart, easily fatigued with poor circulation, and possibly pain in the chest and ribcage area.
Emotional characteristics	These horses are restless, even during rest time or sleep, emotionally detached, and lack concentration.

Jitsu manifestation

Physical characteristics	Constant restlessness, hypersensitivity, nervousness with easy sweating, palpitations and irregular heartbeat. Also, a tendency to diarrhea or constipation.
Emotional characteristics	These horses are restless mentally, hypersensitive, and overreactive emotionally.

Triple Heater Meridian (yang)

Function

Controls spirit and visceral organs circulating energy throughout the body, and supplements the function of the Small Intestine Meridian. Protects the function of the lymphatic system, therefore it protects the entire body. Relates to body heat circulation, controlling thermal regulation. The three 'burning spaces' of Triple Heater relate to respiratory, digestive and elimination organs. Controls circulation to the extremities.

Optimal functioning condition

Physical characteristics

Good adaption to seasonal changes, warming up easily and cooling down quickly after work. Good health, with quick recovery, or no major illnesses.

Emotional characteristics

These horses are even-tempered, not overly excitable or depressive, but have warm, friendly relationships.

Kyo manifestation

Physical characteristics

Weak mucous tissues, nasal problems, a sluggish lymphatic system, sensitivity to humidity and temperature change. A tendency to neck problems accompanied by headaches (including cervical misalignment). Low resistance to colds. Sensitive skin.

Emotional characteristics

These horses are emotionally withdrawn, running hot and cold with unpredictable moods, overly pampered as youngsters and therefore sensitive to changes in the physical environment.

Jitsu manifestation

Physical characteristics

Stiff neck and tight shoulders, lymphatic inflammation, inflammation of mucous membranes, poor circulation, skin problems.

Emotional characteristics

These horses are overcautious, overreact to changes in temperature and environment (cold, heat, humidity) and suffer digestive problems due to nervousness owing to environmental changes.

On the meridian location photographs, the yang meridians are represented by solid lines and the yin meridians are represented by dotted lines. The color representations are the appropriate colors relating to these meridians, except for the Governing and Conception Vessels which have no specific corresponding color and are represented by gray lines. Each of the meridians is bilateral except, again, for the Governing and Conception Vessels which run along the midlines of the horse's body.

LUNG AND LARGE INTESTINE MERIDIANS

The Lung Meridian (yin – white dotted line) surfaces in the chest where it meets the inside of the foreleg near the underarm in the pectoral muscle. It flows upward, slightly toward the outside of the body, then moves down the forearm. It moves down the inside edge of the lower leg, ending slightly above the coronary band. The last point, Lung (Lu) 11, is about two-thirds of the distance from the front of the hoof to the heel.

The Large Intestine Meridian (yang – white solid line) begins at the front inside corner of the foreleg on the coronary band. It then flows up on the inside of the foreleg (approximately center) to the knee. It then crosses laterally over the knee and continues upward, on the outside of the leg, to the elbow, and up the shoulder and across the ventral portion of the neck. It goes along the throat and jaw, and ends at the widest part of the nostril, at Large Intestine (LI) point 20.

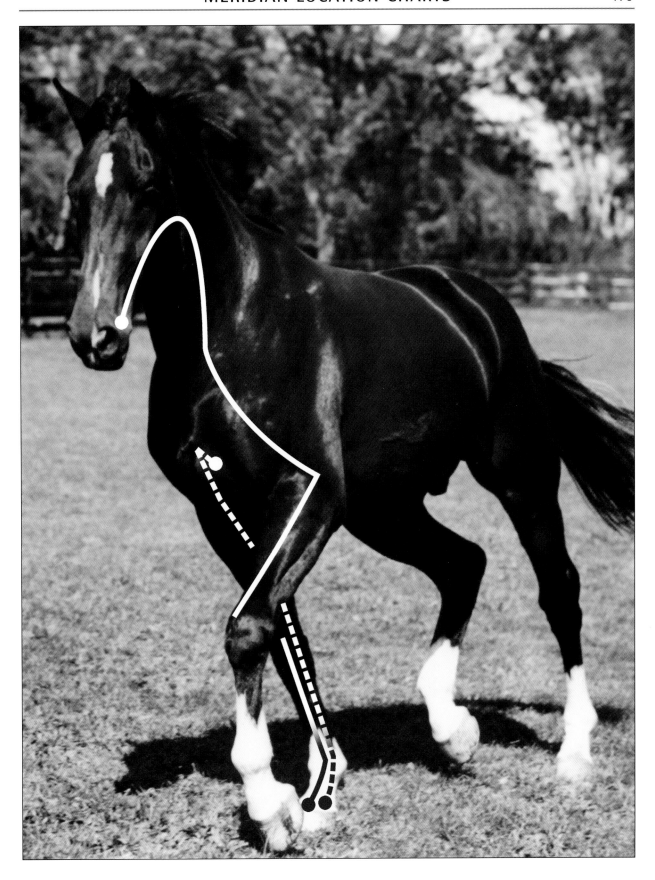

STOMACH AND SPLEEN MERIDIANS

The Stomach Meridian (yang – yellow solid line) begins just below the eye. It moves downward toward the nose, then moves upward along the side of the jawbone. It moves down the neck, below the cervical vertebrae (closer to the midline than Large Intestine Meridian) through the chest and along the lower edge of the abdomen and loins. It flows down the front (slightly to the outside) of the rear leg. It ends at the midline of the coronary band at Stomach (St) point 45.

The Spleen Meridian (yin – yellow dotted line) begins at a point on the inside of the rear leg just above the coronary band, about two-thirds of the way toward the bulb of the heel. It then flows up the inner back side of the pastern. It moves slightly forward as it passes over the inside front of the hock, then goes up the inside center of the leg along the back of the tibia to the stifle, and to a point in front of the tuber coxae. The meridian then runs along the side of the abdomen to the fourth intercostal space, below the level of the point of the shoulder. It then turns and flows toward the hindquarters, and ends approximately at the tenth intercostal space, Spleen (Sp) point 21.

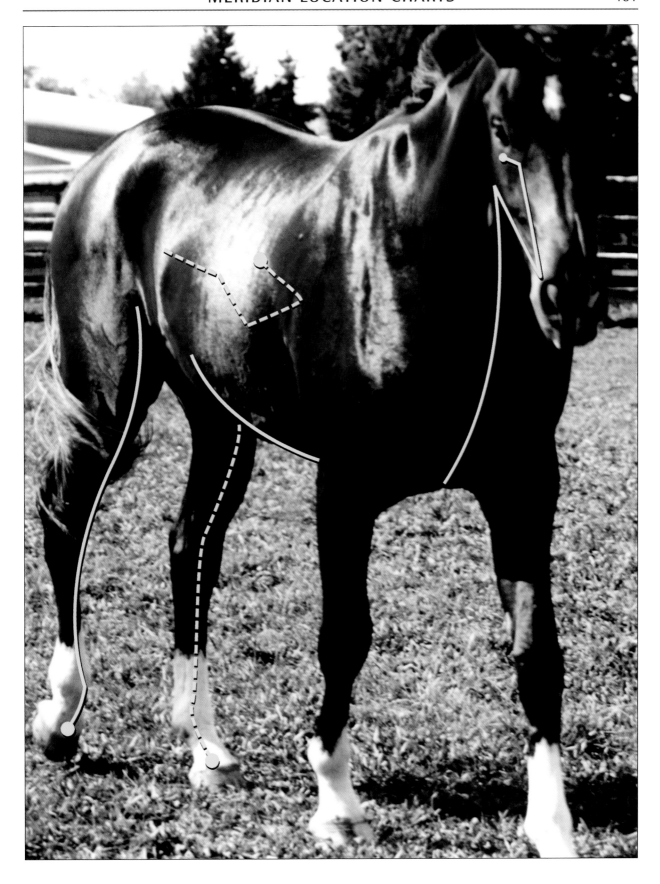

HEART AND SMALL INTESTINE MERIDIANS

The **Heart Meridian** (yin – red dotted line) begins in the armpit, close to the heart. It then goes down the rear portion of the foreleg. At the knee, it crosses and continues down the back edge of the outside portion of the foreleg. It ends at a point one-third of the distance from the heel bulb to the midpoint of the hoof at Heart (Ht) point 9.

The **Small Intestine Meridian** (yang – red solid line) begins at the foot, about one-third the distance from the front of the hoof to the rear. It flows up the outside of the leg, over the pastern and cannon bone, over the knee and goes upward toward the elbow. It moves over the triceps muscle to a point just behind the shoulder joint. It makes two sharp turns in the body of the shoulder, and continues in the neck, crossing the vertebrae and moving to the jaw. It ends at Small Intestine (SI) point 19 on the outside of the base of the ear.

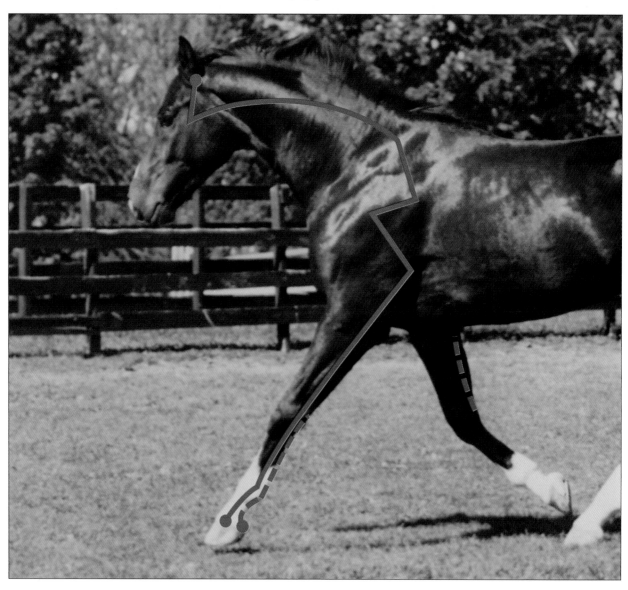

BLADDER AND KIDNEY MERIDIANS

The **Bladder Meridian** (yang – blue solid line) begins at the inner corner of the eye and goes upward and over the poll. It moves down the neck about two to three finger-widths from the base of the mane. At the withers, it splits into two branches. The two lines are parallel to the spine. The upper branch is two to four finger-widths from the center line of the spine, the lower branch about three to five finger-widths lower. The double channel becomes one line near the tail and continues to move down the leg in the crease of the biceps femoris and the semitendinosus muscles. It continues down the outside of the leg and ends at Bladder (Bl) point 67, which is about two-thirds the distance from the front to the back of the hoof.

The **Kidney Meridian** (yin – blue dotted line) begins at the coronary band on the hind leg at the point just between the bulbs of the heels. It then travels up the inside rear portion of the hind leg to the hock. It makes a clockwise circle and continues up the inside of the leg to the groin area. It continues along the abdomen, approximately two to three inches from the midline, goes to the chest and ends between the breastbone and first rib, at Kidney (K) point 27.

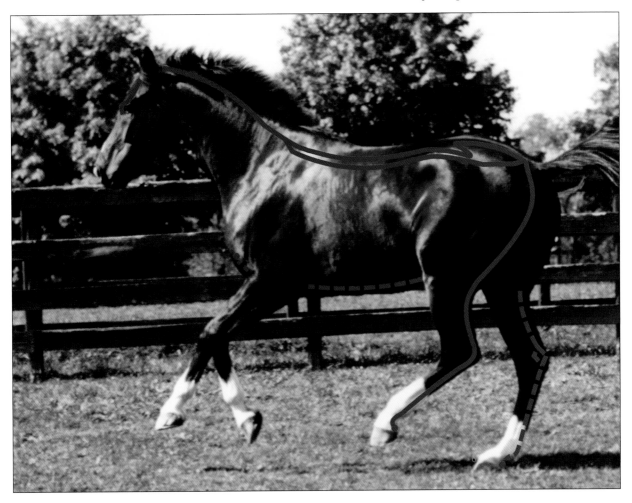

HEART CONSTRICTOR AND TRIPLE HEATER MERIDIANS

The Heart Constrictor Meridian, (yin – red dotted line) also called the Pericardium Meridian, begins deep inside the body at the sac that surrounds the heart. It surfaces in the space between the fifth and sixth ribs, near the inside of the upper leg. It then moves down the middle of the inside of the foreleg toward the chestnut, going towards the back side of the knee. It moves toward the back inside of the lower leg (along the flexor tendon) and down to the middle of the bulbs of the heel at Heart Constrictor (HC) point 9. Technically, it ends on the bottom of the hoof, in the frog but, for accessibility, the point between the bulbs can be used as an ending point.

The Triple Heater Meridian (yang – red solid line) begins at the mid-point of the coronary band on the foreleg. It continues up the pastern and cannon bone to the knee, and continues up the outside of the upper leg, about midway between the front and back of the foreleg. It moves toward the elbow, and along the back side of the humerus to the shoulder joint. It then crosses the scapula and continues along the neck, below the vertebrae, above the Large Intestine Meridian. It goes to the ear and ends at the outside end of the eyebrow at Triple Heater (TH) point 23.

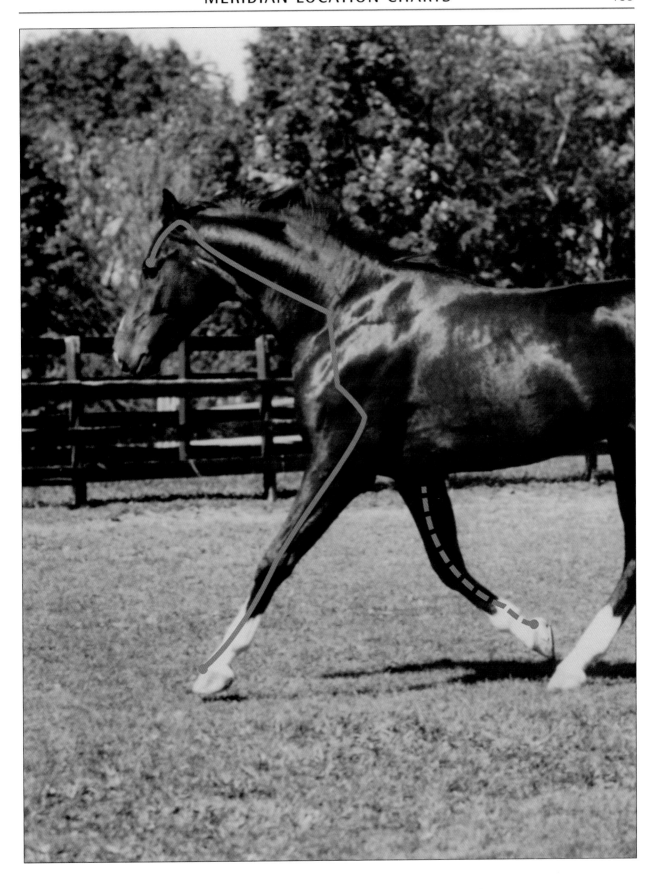

GALL BLADDER AND LIVER MERIDIANS

The Gall Bladder Meridian (yang – green solid line) begins at the outer corner of the eye, it moves upward toward the poll and then down the neck (just below the Bladder Meridian) to the middle of the scapula. Here it enters the chest cavity and flows through the abdomen. It resurfaces and travels up to Gall Bladder (GB) point 25, which is on the outside of the last rib. It moves upward toward the pelvic area, then downward below the point of the hip to the hip joint. It then passes through the mid portion of the hindquarters and down the middle of the outside of the rear leg, to Gall Bladder (GB) point 44, which is on the coronary band about one-third of the distance from the front to the back of the hoof.

The Liver Meridian (yin – green dotted line) begins at the point just above the coronary band on the inside rear leg, about one-third of the distance from the middle of the front hoof wall to the heel. It then travels up the middle of the inside of the rear leg, flowing over the pastern and cannon bone where it moves toward the front of the leg slightly as it passes over the hock and up the femur. The Liver Meridian enters the pubic area and travels forward toward the head. The meridian slants downward and ends at Liver (Li) point 14, which is located in the space between the thirteenth and fourteenth ribs, at about the level of the elbow.

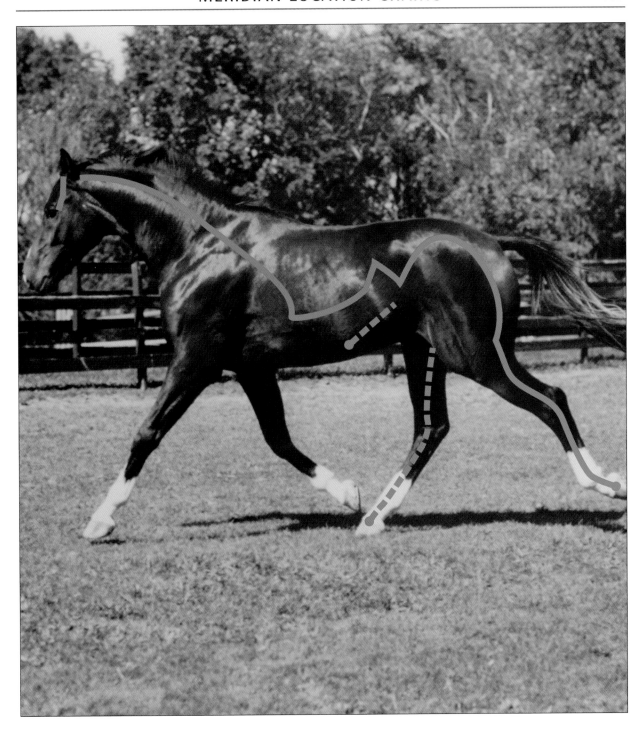

**CONCEPTION VESSEL
AND GOVERNING VESSEL**

The Conception Vessel (yin – gray* broken line) travels the full length of the body along the ventral midline. It begins at a point below the anus and runs between the hind legs through the genitals and umbilicus, continuing along the midline of the abdomen and through the chest, passing up the midline along the neck and head. It ends at Conception Vessel (CV) point 24, which is on the lower lip. Please note that this vessel is not bilateral.

The Governing Vessel (yang – gray* solid line) starts in a depression between the anus and the root of the tail. It moves toward the head along the dorsal midline of the back, and runs over the top of the head and face and ends at a point between the upper lip and gums, Governing Vessel (GV) point 28.

*Where the lines on the photo are white instead of gray, the channel goes along the midline between the ears and under the tail (Governing Vessel) and between the front and back legs (Conception Vessel).

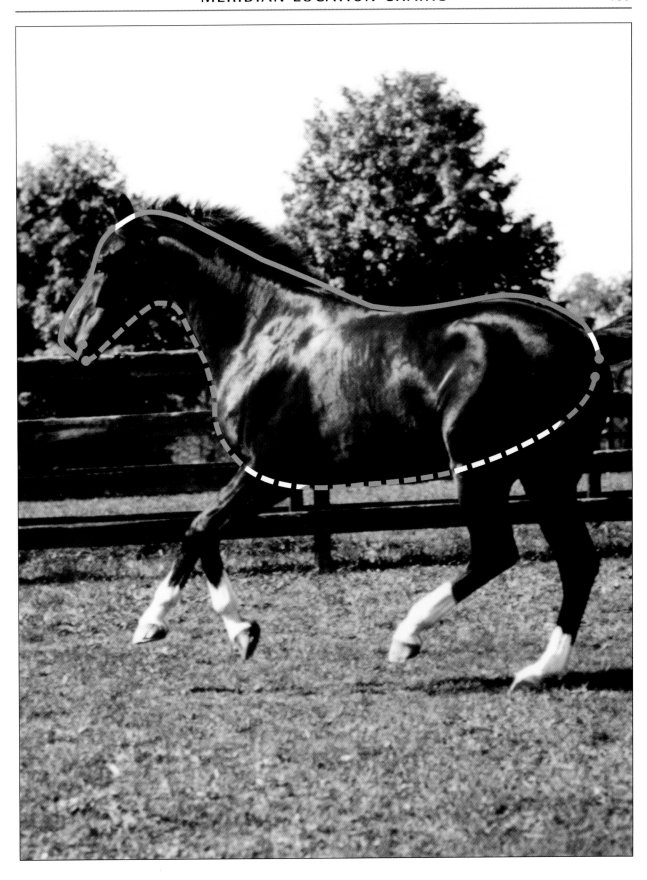

INTRODUCTION

I had been doing shiatsu with horses for about two years before I ever saw a chart of equine acupuncture points or meridian lines. This was to my advantage; the time allowed me to develop my intuition and the sensitivity in my hands. I felt for meridian lines based on what I knew of human locations and the imbalances I felt while touching, as well as what I saw during visual observation. Finally, a vet gave me a copy of Westermeyer's book on acupoints. The book was occasionally helpful for specific physiological conditions.

In 1985, in my new neighbourhood in New Jersey, I was travelling around with a vet for the purpose of making contacts and learning. He asked if I might be able to help an ex-racehorse (a syndicated stallion valued at six million dollars). The horse had a low sperm count and was suffering a loss of desire. I had no idea if I could help and was not given the opportunity to establish any rapport with the horse who was unruly and looked dangerous as he was led in by someone who resembled the Incredible Hulk. The horse snorted and stomped restlessly as I looked in Westermeyer's book and found a few points for impotence. I tentatively reached out and held these points. The 'treatment' took less than five minutes. I felt frustrated, perhaps having taken on the horse's predominant characteristic.

A week or so later the vet saw me and said 'Hannay, your timing was immaculate. His sperm count went up and his desire has returned'. I asked that his next foal be named after me.

I do not know if I helped the horse but as a first foray into using points for specific problems, it was an impressive lesson.

Since then I have seen many charts, from ancient Chinese charts to modern renditions of lines and points. I particularly like *Equine Acupressure* by Nancy Zidonis, Amy Snow and Marie Soderberg and *Equine Atlas of Acupuncture Loci* by Peggy Fleming DVM. The point location charts in the following pages have been reproduced from this latter title by kind permission of Dr. Fleming. (Please note that any point or terms on these charts not mentioned in my text are references to Chinese acupuncture.)

Please understand that shiatsu is not a point-to-point system, or a button-pushing exercise. Use the charts as a guide but remember that we are dealing with energy, and the nature of energy is change. You may feel a particular meridian in a slightly different place from one day to the next. Points that require pressure will make themselves apparent to you when there is an imbalance.

In my courses I do not teach points or meridian location until Levels 2 and 3. I know it is more important for students to learn to feel energy flow through their hands before turning the work into an intellectual exercise. Students who are too concerned with points have problems trusting their instincts and letting the joy of following energy during the session guide them.

I think of a meridian line as a channel of many points, some of which manifest themselves during times of physical and/or mental distress. These points may pull you in with the desire to be held, or push you away without needing further stimulation.

The meridians relate to organ function more than to the actual organ. For example, horses do not have gall bladders but they do have biliary systems. The Gall Bladder Meridian represents this function. Incorporating meridian work with body movement exercises will help you work with a well-rounded approach.

In traditional Chinese theory, each meridian has a specific direction of energy flow. In the front legs, yin meridians flow toward the feet and the yang meridians flow from the feet upward. In the back legs, the yin meridians begin in the feet and flow upward, and the yang meridians flow downward to the feet.

In general, I like to follow the Masanuga approach: energy flows outward from the center of the body toward the extremities. I work intuitively, case by case, letting the energy express itself to me and show me the direction it wants to go in order to rebalance itself.

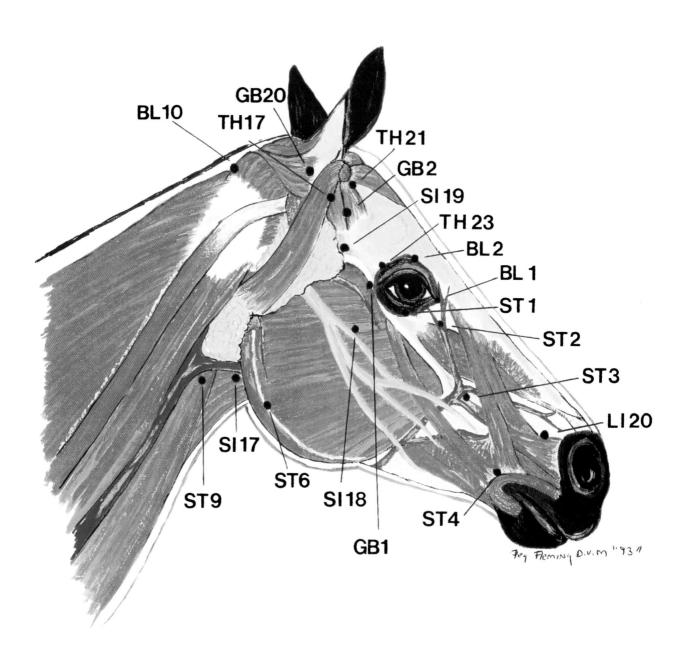

BL10
GB20
TH17
TH21
GB2
SI19
TH23
BL2
BL1
ST1
ST2
ST3
LI20
SI17
ST6
SI18
ST9
GB1
ST4

Peg Fleming D.V.M "93"

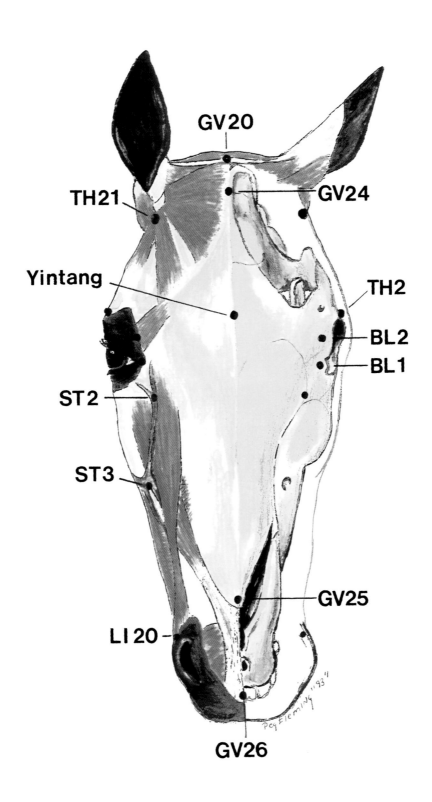

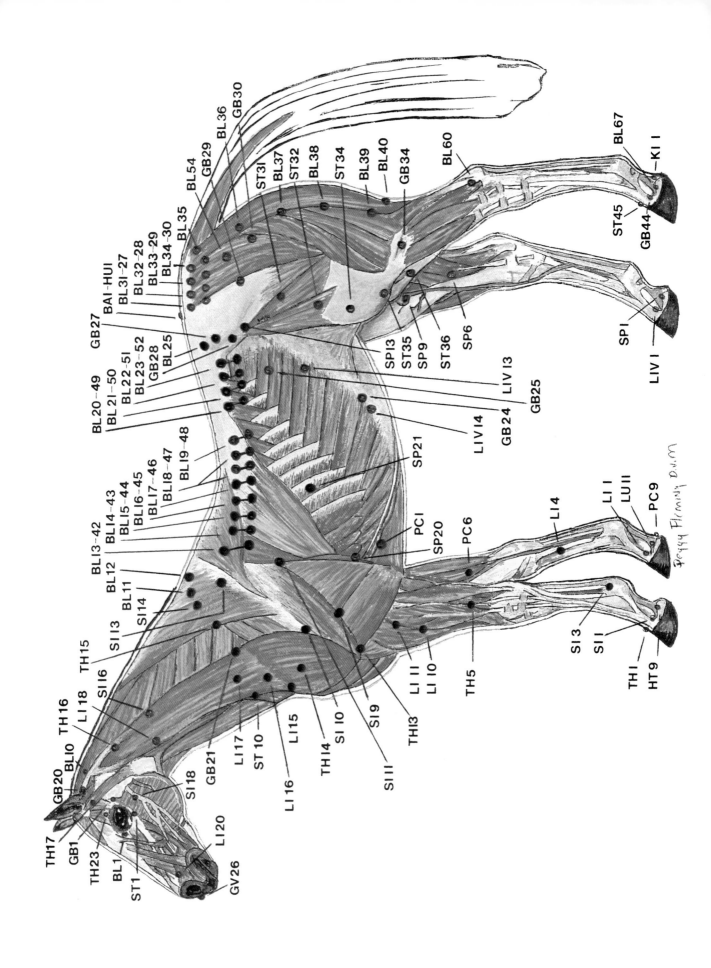

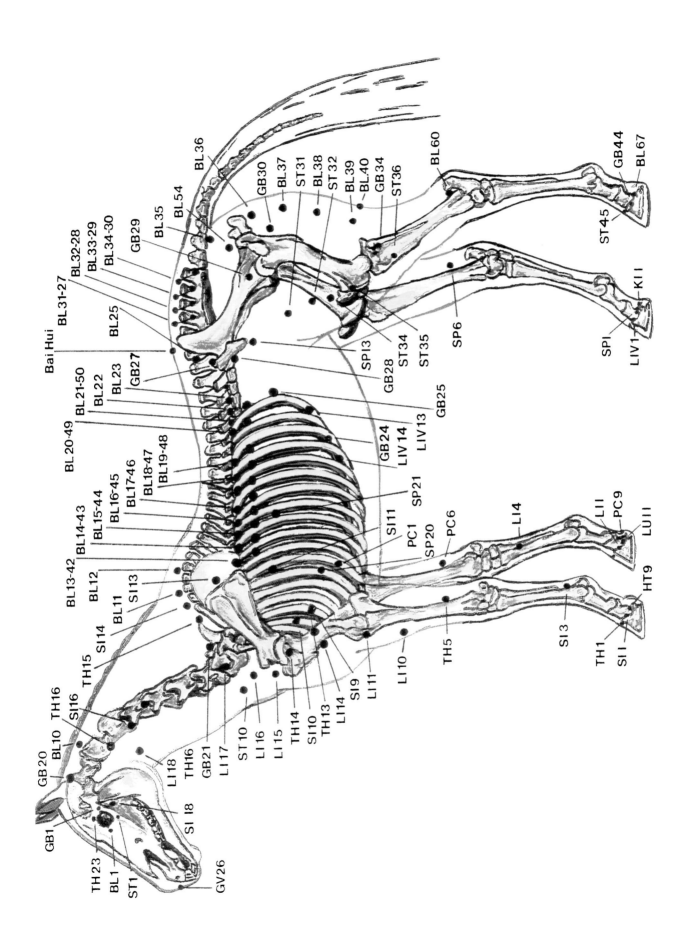

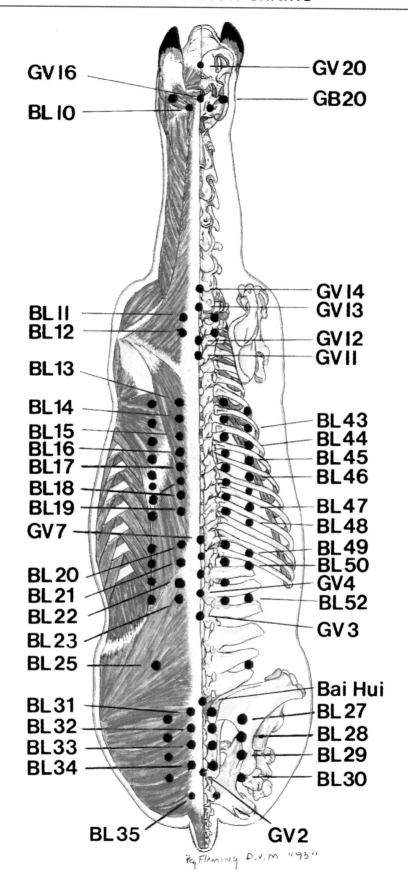

GV16
GV20
BL10
GB20

GV14
GV13
BL11
BL12
GV12
GV11

BL13

BL14
BL43
BL15
BL44
BL16
BL45
BL17
BL46
BL18
BL19
BL47
GV7
BL48
BL49
BL20
BL50
BL21
GV4
BL22
BL52
BL23
GV3

BL25

Bai Hui
BL31
BL27
BL32
BL28
BL33
BL29
BL34
BL30

BL35
GV2

Peg Fleming D.V.m "93"

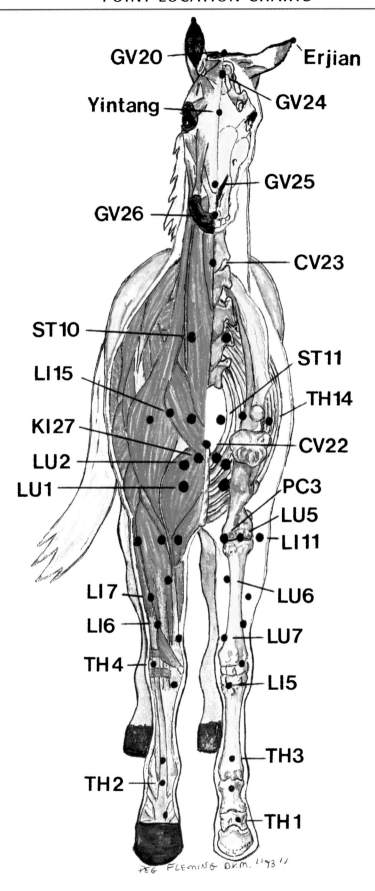

GV20

Yintang

GV26

ST10

LI15

KI27

LU2

LU1

LI7

LI6

TH4

TH2

Erjian

GV24

GV25

CV23

ST11

TH14

CV22

PC3

LU5

LI11

LU6

LU7

LI5

TH3

TH1

PEG FLEMING D.V.M. 1193

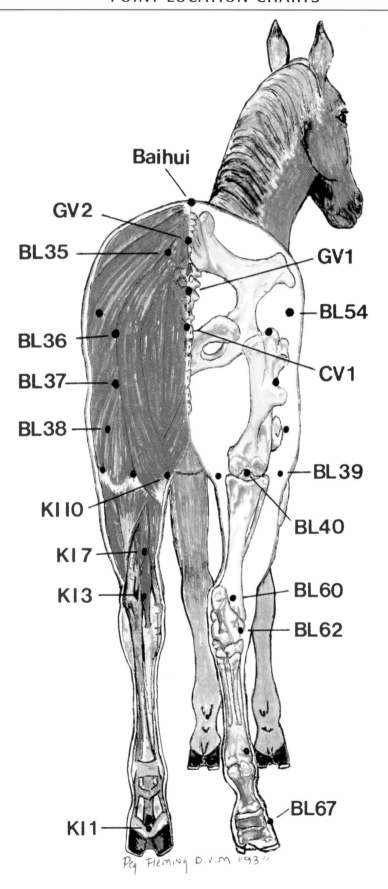

Baihui

GV 2

BL 35

GV 1

BL 54

BL 36

CV 1

BL 37

BL 38

BL 39

KI 10

BL 40

KI 7

BL 60

KI 3

BL 62

BL 67

KI 1

Peg Fleming D.V.M "93"

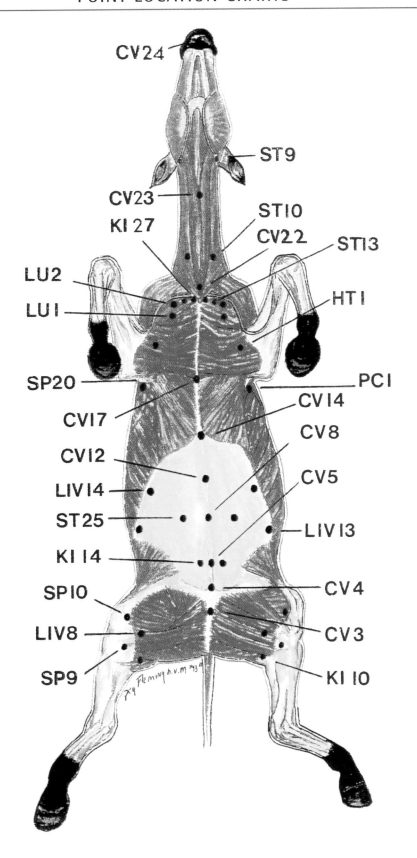

FRONT LIMB

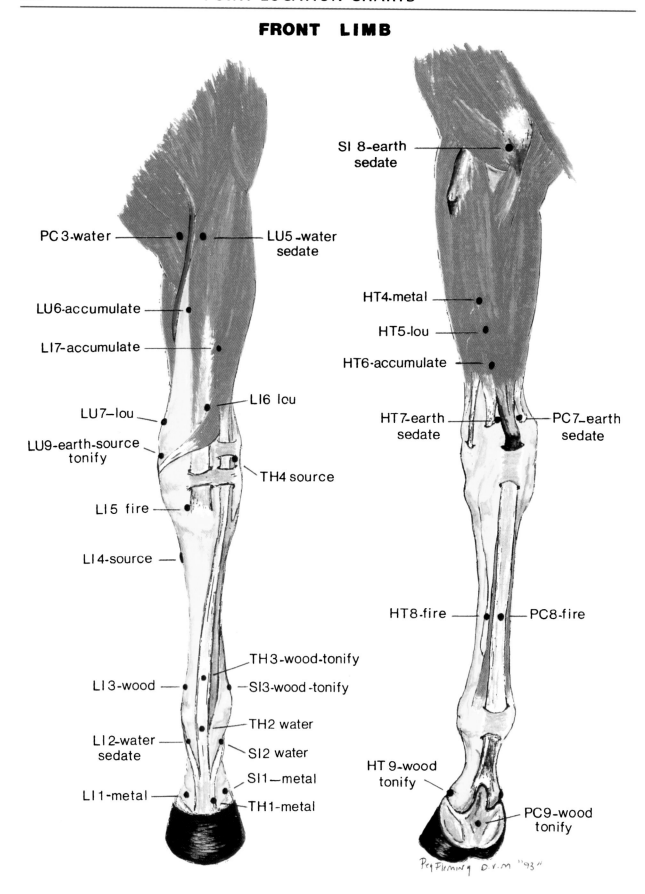

PC 3-water

LU5 -water
sedate

LU6-accumulate

LI7-accumulate

LU7—lou

LI6 lou

LU9-earth-source
tonify

TH4 source

LI5 fire

LI4-source

TH3-wood-tonify

LI3-wood

SI3-wood -tonify

TH2 water

LI2-water
sedate

SI2 water

SI1—metal

LI1-metal

TH1-metal

SI 8-earth
sedate

HT4-metal

HT5-lou

HT6-accumulate

HT7-earth
sedate

PC 7-earth
sedate

HT8-fire

PC8-fire

HT 9-wood
tonify

PC9-wood
tonify

Peg Fleming D.V.M "93"

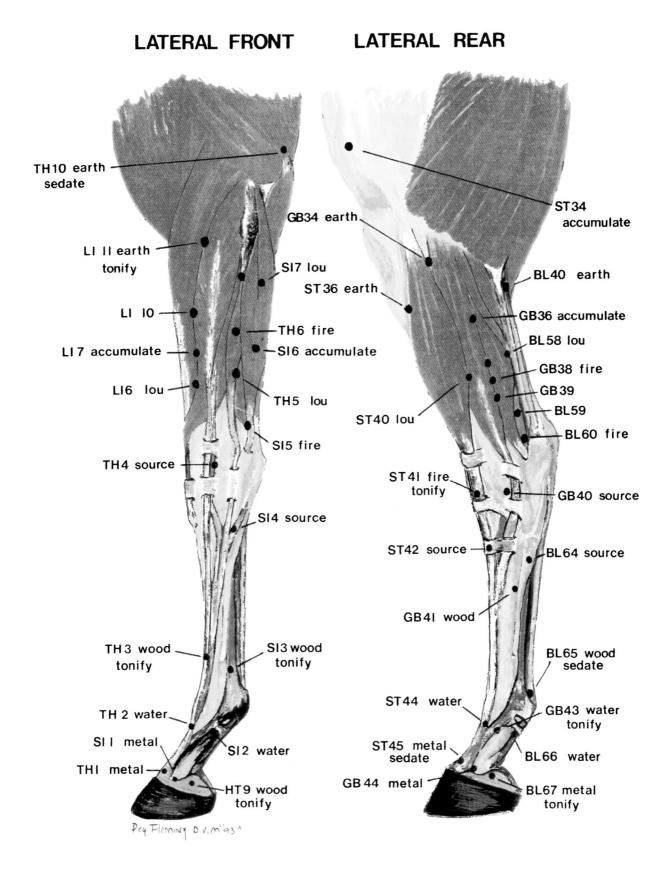

LATERAL FRONT

TH10 earth
sedate

LI II earth
tonify

GB34 earth

SI7 lou

LI 10

ST36 earth

LI7 accumulate

TH6 fire

LI6 lou

SI6 accumulate

TH5 lou

SI5 fire

TH4 source

SI4 source

TH3 wood
tonify

SI3 wood
tonify

TH2 water

SI1 metal

THI metal

SI2 water

HT9 wood
tonify

LATERAL REAR

ST34
accumulate

BL40 earth

GB36 accumulate

BL58 lou

GB38 fire

GB39

BL59

BL60 fire

ST40 lou

ST41 fire
tonify

GB40 source

ST42 source

BL64 source

GB41 wood

BL65 wood
sedate

ST44 water

GB43 water
tonify

ST45 metal
sedate

BL66 water

GB44 metal

BL67 metal
tonify

Peg Fleming D.V.m'93"

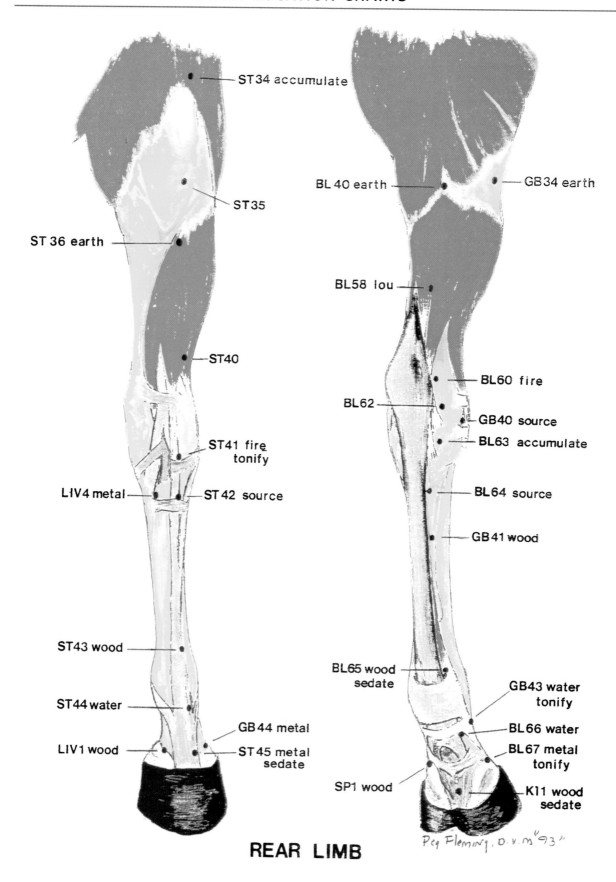

ST34 accumulate

ST35

ST 36 earth

ST40

ST41 fire
tonify

LIV4 metal — ST 42 source

ST43 wood

ST44 water

LIV1 wood

GB44 metal

ST 45 metal
sedate

BL 40 earth — GB34 earth

BL58 lou

BL60 fire

BL62

GB40 source

BL63 accumulate

BL64 source

GB41 wood

BL65 wood
sedate

GB43 water
tonify

BL66 water

BL67 metal
tonify

SP1 wood

K11 wood
sedate

Peg Fleming, D.v.m "93"

REAR LIMB

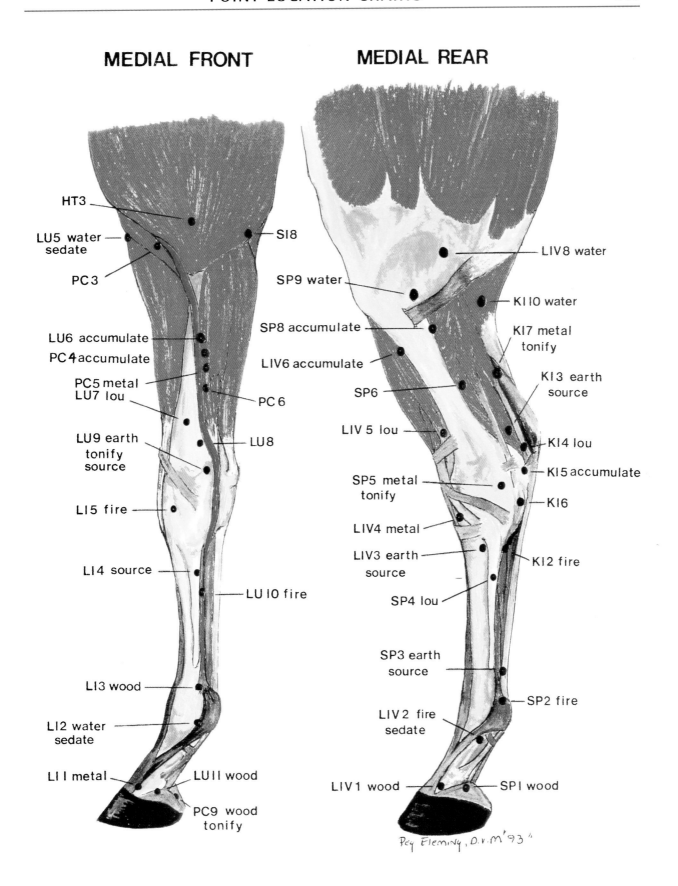

MEDIAL FRONT

HT3
LU5 water sedate
PC3
LU6 accumulate
PC4 accumulate
PC5 metal
LU7 lou
LU9 earth tonify source
LI5 fire
LI4 source
LI3 wood
LI2 water sedate
LI1 metal
SI8
PC6
LU8
LU10 fire
LU11 wood
PC9 wood tonify

MEDIAL REAR

LIV8 water
SP9 water
KI10 water
SP8 accumulate
KI7 metal tonify
LIV6 accumulate
KI3 earth source
SP6
LIV5 lou
KI4 lou
KI5 accumulate
SP5 metal tonify
KI6
LIV4 metal
LIV3 earth source
KI2 fire
SP4 lou
SP3 earth source
SP2 fire
LIV2 fire sedate
LIV1 wood
SP1 wood

Peg Fleming, D.v.m '93

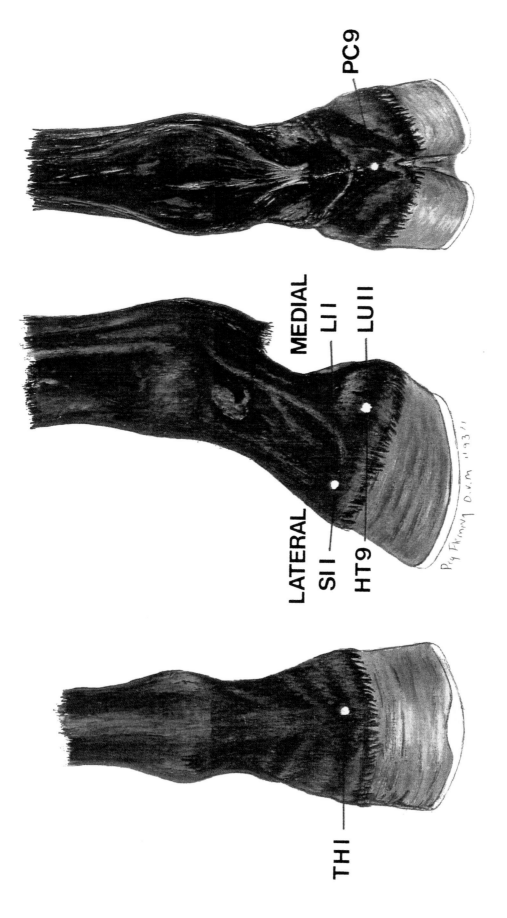

PC9

MEDIAL
LI I
LU I I

LATERAL
S I I
HT9

Pq Farang D.v.m 1'93''

TH I

TING POINTS OF THE FRONT HOOF

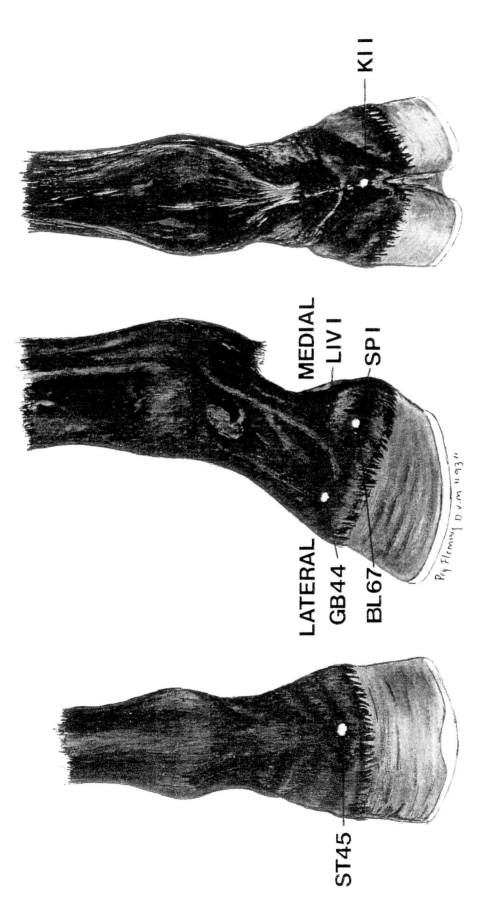

K1 1

MEDIAL
LIV 1
SP 1

LATERAL
GB44
BL67

Pcq Fleming D.V.M "93"

ST45

TING POINTS OF THE REAR HOOF

ASSOCIATED POINTS

How to use the associated points

When working on the Bladder Meridian, you may find one or many sensitive points. If the area is bilaterally painful, you may ascertain the meridian the area is associated with by checking the point locations charts. The associated points are called *yu* points. Check the associated meridian for sensitivity, sensitive areas, kyo and jitsu. For example, the Lung Meridian diagnostic area may be sensitive. If you know your horse has allergies, catches cold easily, or has had lung-related problems, it will not be unusual for this area to be sensitive. Remember that the associated points are bilateral. Do not base your observations *only* on the associated points. We are looking at the entire individual.

The associated points

Bladder 13	Lung	8th intercostal space (between 7th and 8th thoracic vertebrae)
Bladder 14	Heart Constrictor	9th intercostal space (between 8th and 9th thoracic vertebrae)
Bladder 15	Heart	10th intercostal space
Bladder 18	Liver	13th and 14th intercostal spaces
Bladder 19	Gall Bladder	15th intercostal space
Bladder 20	Spleen	17th intercostal space
Bladder 21	Stomach	3 cun* lateral to the midline, just caudal to the last rib
Bladder 22	Triple Heater	between 1st and 2nd lumbar vertebrae
Bladder 23	Kidney	between 2nd and 3rd lumbar vertebrae
Bladder 25	Large Intestine	between 5th and 6th lumbar vertebrae
Bladder 27	Small Intestine	between 1st and 2nd sacral vertebrae
Bladder 28	Bladder	between 2nd and 3rd sacral vertebrae

*Unit of measurement, usually about three fingers width.

Part V

TREATMENT ADVICE
AND PROCEDURES

Evaluating the Horse to Ascertain Appropriate Procedures

First, I must mention that when observing a horse, I look at wholeness. One of my early teachers, Shinmai Kishi, said, 'look for the blue sky'. I see the horse in a positive way. I look at what is right with him before looking for what is wrong. I always find something to give a compliment for. Do not get into the habit of seeing negativity. See the blue sky.

After meeting the horse, or greeting one already known, I ask the owner to walk him, or perhaps even trot him a bit. I center myself and quiet my breathing. I walk behind the horse and imitate his walk. I move my shoulders and arms as he moves his shoulders and front legs. I get my own neck and head moving a bit as well. I move my legs and hips in as close an approximation of the horse's legs and hips as possible. At these times I always wish I had a tail. I walk alongside him to observe shoulder movement. I walk backwards in front of him to see him walking toward me. I listen to the rhythm of his footfalls. I look at everything, including tracking and inward or outward swing of feet and legs. I look for an uneven rise and fall of the muscles of the hindquarters, a lack of undulation of muscles, how he is using the energy of his muscles and meridians and if he is propelling himself from the rear or pulling himself along. I look for areas of kyo and jitsu in areas of the body as well as within the meridian locations. I see whether or not he feels connected to his own body as a unit, or simply a conglomeration of separate parts. Am I comfortable in my own body as I mimic his? Am I happy inside and pain free? This technique gives me a picture of wholeness, as well as imperfection. I also look at his conformation to determine what type of problems he might be prone to. His conformation gives me a good idea of what I may expect to accomplish based on his physical limitations and attributes.

When practicing this technique, try to walk behind as many horses as possible with few or no glaring problems so that you can understand what is right before looking for what is wrong.

All sessions no matter how short should begin and end with all-over stroking.

THE FOAL AND THE YOUNG HORSE

To young horses, everything is new and exciting. Their energy is jumping and seemingly endless, until they suddenly collapse into sleep. These babies react to a shiatsu session as a normal part of everything they learn each day. They are not surprised by the sensations of moving energy in their bodies, or surprised by the feelings of relaxation that come during and after a treatment. These relaxation responses may be similar to the feeling of recently being fed by mother and sedated by the calcium in her milk.

Keep the foal's session time short and leave him wanting more, rather than wandering away from you, bored. Try to work on him without restraint, so he has the choice of having you work on him or not. He may present you with the places where he most wants to be touched. You may be working on him as he moves about, which is fine, as long as he is enjoying himself. Let him express himself during the session. Ongoing shiatsu will help a foal or young horse to grow mentally as well as be comfortable physically during the demands of being trained for work. Injuries may be unheard of as he grows into adulthood, and the consistent shiatsu gives him the added benefit of understanding his body in a special way as he grows up.

The foal's body is usually so flexible that it does not need stretching for the purpose of increasing range of motion. Stretch him only to the point of resistance, or less, to educate you both about his body's capacity and to keep energy moving. Vary your sessions to keep both of you interested. Work with a spirit of fun and laughter.

Working with foals and young horses helps encourage the bond between horse and human. It will also make weaning less stressful; work on the foal for at least a few minutes each day for the week leading up to weaning, and each day for the week following, in addition to regular treatments.

In general, a good idea for session procedure might be five minutes on the back each day or every other day for about four treatments. Work only with the palms as fingertips may be too specific. Then, increase the session time by a minute or so and work on the hindquarters with your palms and add a leg jiggle if he is resting his leg. Then, try working only on the feet and possibly the tail for a few treatments. Add foot rotations only if he is secure standing on three legs for a short time. Sometimes you will only work on the face and ears for a few minutes. Work with the foal in the spirit of exploration and joy!

PREGNANT MARES

During the time leading up to breeding, it may be helpful to work on your mare. The treatments will help energy to flow, especially to the reproductive organs. Work on Conception Vessel, Kidney, Stomach and Spleen Meridians.

During gestation time you may keep working on a mare, however, avoid too many stretches on yin type mares (delicate, slender, long boned, temperamental). Concentrate on meridians, like Bladder and Kidney, and Heart Constrictor. Yang type mares can tolerate a more active session. Avoid working on Spleen 6, Stomach 36 and Bladder 60 on any pregnant mare, although these points may be helpful during labor. Regular sessions will keep you in contact with her in a way that will immediately alert you to any changes the vet may need to know about. It will also help her to deliver more comfortably. You may assist the birth process by giving shiatsu on the yin meridians of the rear legs, and Bladder Meridian on the back. Also work on the ears to stimulate energy throughout the entire body. Work strongly on Spleen 6, Stomach 36 and Bladder 60.

Following delivery, help her to recover her energy with frequent sessions. These may be short with the frequent demands of motherhood. Work on Stomach, Gall Bladder, Bladder and Kidney Meridians, and be prepared for a very interested foal trying to get your attention. Keep your movements slow and deliberate.

Working on mares following delivery while they are nursing will help them maintain their energy during the tremendous demands of this time. It will also keep the bond between you strong. Mares who receive shiatsu while having a foal at their side also tend to be more sociable with their human visitors.

OLDER HORSES

With the problems of age, such as worn and aching joints, muscular changes, and going from a life of activity to relative inactivity, the older horse is a prime candidate for shiatsu. Most older horses should have some little job to do, for psychological and physical wellbeing, and they should enjoy the company of other horses, rather than being turned out alone.

The first time an older horse receives shiatsu, he may look very surprised. He may think he has experienced everything there is to experience in life. The sensations of the session are so new and wonderful that he may behave in a somewhat uncharacteristic manner as a result.

Regular sessions on a horse who is older, but still working, will keep him going more comfortably and possibly for a longer period of time. You will understand his body as it ages and be able to respond to these changes. A full body session each week is suggested, but two shorter sessions are fine too. If possible, do the preride and postride treatment each time he is about to be worked.

Begin with very simple and short sessions to accustom the horse to treatment. Concentrate on techniques that require movement, such as foot and leg rotations, stretches and jiggles. Work on Gall Bladder and Liver Meridians as these have a relationship with the muscles, tendons and ligaments. Work the ears to improve digestion, elimination and energy flow throughout the body.

Retired horses may not seem to need treatments since they are turned out to pasture and look relaxed and content but shiatsu sessions every week or two (or more often if possible) will be a nice way to say thank you for years of hard work. It will also keep the retiree healthy and happy for years to come and will possibly extend life expectancy.

Work on small rotations and regular stretching done slowly, especially the neck. Work on Lung and Large Intestine Meridians, as well as any others you may choose. Let your horse express his needs to you and listen carefully. The retired horse has a lot of time to think about things.

DRESSAGE HORSES

This sophisticated dancer needs regular shiatsu to keep him from straining muscles whether from learning new lessons or performing. The angles of their movements require some specific techniques. For example, when stretching the front leg forward, also stretch it to each side. This may be done by beginning with a long forward stretch, releasing it a bit, taking it outward, releasing a bit, and stretching it toward the other leg.

The upper leg diagonal stretch (*see* page 86), will stretch his upper leg and shoulder diagonally in each direction. Hold these stretches for several seconds and always release slowly. When stretching the rear legs, stretch the leg straight back, and then augment it by stretching it away from the other back leg, and then toward the other back leg, releasing it slightly each time between each movement, (*see* Meridian Stretches on pages 102–3). Work the feet, incorporating stretches into the rotations. Be sure to do neck work, especially the lengthening stretches. Tail work will be beneficial and may improve tail carriage during performance.

With any show horse, you may not want to work on them immediately before, or even the same day as, the show. They may become too relaxed when you need them to be psyched up. Certainly, give them a mini session after they are cooled down, and a full body session the next day.

As a beginning practitioner of shiatsu for horses, I worked on a horse and rider a few hours before a big dressage test, resulting in both horse and rider being too mellow. They spent their time enjoying the music and the sunlight and forgetting the test. Their instructor was less than pleased with all of us. For the horse and rider, it was the loveliest time they had ever had in the show arena. I enjoyed their performance immensely.

SHOWJUMPERS

With the tremendous effort of take-off, sailing through the air, and concussion of landing, the jumper is particularly at risk of injury. Because of its association with impetus, the Bladder Meridian is a particularly important one to incorporate into any session for the jumper. Consider the need for spring in the rear legs, as well as the force of landing, from a height, on the front legs.

For the rear legs, in addition to rotation and stretches, I recommend holding the leg in rotation position, and lifting it straight up to compress momentarily the joints of hip, stifle, hock and fetlock. Release the leg directly down into a neutral position, then lift it again and release it so that the foot, still in the air, is slightly in a rearward position. Repeat this sequence three to five times. Do foot rotations, and include the stretch position that stretches the front of the fetlock joint (Stomach Meridian in this area). Hold this stretch for ten to fifteen seconds.

For the front legs and shoulders, do several small rotations, and very gradually build to larger ones. Small rotations particularly target, and let you become aware of, the condition of the joints. During the rotations, concentrate on the rearward movement of the leg, as this will help release tension in the chest. Work on the chest area and on the meridians under the neck (Stomach and Large Intestine). With the front leg still lifted, bend the knee so the fetlock joint comes as close to the leg as possible, without actually bending the fetlock joint to accomplish this. Hold for a few seconds and release. Do this knee exercise three to five times slowly. The foot rotations and stretches will also be helpful. These exercises are particularly important since the impact of landing can cause so much stress to the entire front part of the body of the jumper. Do all the techniques for the shoulder.

WESTERN HORSES

Western show riding incorporates a lot of spins, turns, sudden stops from high speed, and shifts of body-weight. Sometimes during a tight turn, the horse looks like his side is actually touching the ground. There is a lot of stress on the joints, particularly the shoulder joints and muscles.

A working ranch horse must know his job very well and be able to make decisions quickly and respond in a flash when herding animals, cutting one from the herd, or coming upon a dangerous situation outside the ranch. They need gentle work to release tired, strained and possibly overworked muscles. Small rotations, gradually becoming full rotations, will help ease tired joints and muscles. Work Small Intestine Meridian in the shoulders. Do not overstretch tired muscles. Work on Gall Bladder Meridian (for its association with the decision making process) and Liver Meridian (for muscles, tendons, and ligaments), Kidney and Bladder, and Triple Heater. Do all the shoulder work slowly, changing often from side to side to avoid the horse standing on three legs for too long.

VAULTING HORSES

The patience of these marvelous horses, who go around and around endlessly while children of all sizes, and small adults, leap on and off their backs in various combinations of groupings, amazes me. They take care of their people so beautifully with steady movement and subtle balance changes.

Vaulting horses are usually heavily muscled stocky horses. Their working stride and movements are pretty limited so they would benefit from any shiatsu technique you choose to do. Keep your sessions varied and interesting; in general, rotations, stretches and neck work would be of benefit to the vaulting horse. Neck stretches that lengthen will ease a neck that is bent slightly as they always work in a circle. Work on the withers and the hindquarters in particular and work extensively on the Bladder Meridian in the back.

DRIVING HORSES

Horses that pull weight take a lot of strain in the shoulders, front legs and even the neck. Since there is more pull than pushing-from-behind action you may help them by doing all the shoulder work, front leg rotations and stretches, and neck techniques. The hindquarters may need slow tonification work, to energize the area and keep the horse aware of the power in the rear of his body. Work the Small Intestine Meridian in the shoulder.

Specific Conditions

These techniques are not intended to replace proper diagnosis and appropriate treatment by a veterinarian and/or farrier.

LAMENESS – FINDING THE PROBLEM AND ADDRESSING IT AT THE SAME TIME

Observe your horse and imitate and evaluate his movements as explained on page 208. Following this movement evaluation, I then relax my eyes and scan the body on each side. Many times my relaxed eyes get 'pulled' somewhere. I have often found this is the area of disturbance. Keep this area in mind as you begin your techniques but avoid working on it at the beginning of the session. If you are not certain where the problem is following this visual observation, proceed with the general session outlines below. (When energy is exactly where it is supposed to be, it does not feel like anything very interesting or noteworthy but when it is misplaced, unbalanced or sick, it becomes interesting, palpable and observable. It is this misplaced energy that we look for which will help us to understand how an imbalance manifests itself in the body.)

I learned I had the ability to find the painful area at a glance many years ago. I was working with the US Equestrian Team during a three-day event. During a break, I was walking the cross-country course when I came upon a woman walking her horse, one of the entries. We struck up a conversation that began with me saying what a beautiful horse she had. As I looked at him, my eyes immediately went to a section of his hindquarters as his owner began to tell me that he was a bit off occasionally, but the problem was not glaring enough to find, or to keep him out of competition. I took a risk and said, 'it's there', pointing to the area near his stifle where my eyes had been drawn. She looked at me quizzically and said that is what she had suspected but the vet could not find anything. I then introduced myself. She started to laugh, saying a friend had suggested she contact me when she was in New Jersey (she lived out of state). There we were, in the middle of a huge field, destined to meet for the sake of her horse.

When looking for the causes of lameness, begin with the Bladder Meridian along the back and back of the legs. You may find some sensitive places that relate to the problem. Work the kyo and jitsu places gently. Bladder Meridian in the leg helps the leg to move forward, so pay attention to areas of stiffness there. Work deeply on the hindquarters if the horse is able to tolerate it, otherwise work more superficially to begin with and work into deeper pressure. Then work on the leg meridians. Gall Bladder and Liver Meridians are good choices because of their relationship with the muscles, tendons, and ligaments. Work Kidney Meridian for its relationship with the joints. Work Stomach Meridian because it is so involved with rearward movement of the leg, as well as drawing it forward. On the front legs, work Small Intestine Meridian and Large Intestine Meridian, for their location more than their function. Working meridians will get energy moving in preparation for rotations.

In shiatsu, treatment is diagnosis and diagnosis is treatment, so your sleuthing is very productive. Begin with foot rotations, going slowly, noticing exactly what meridians are being stretched as you go around in your circle. Note that small rotations teach you about the condition of the joints, so concentrate on small rotations first. Larger rotations show you the condition of the muscles. For example, if the front area is tight, Large Intestine may be restricted. After foot rotations, begin leg rotations, not keeping your horse standing on any three legs for too long. If rotations seem fluid, begin to systematically stretch the limbs. Then, work on the Bladder Meridian again, beginning with the neck. Do some gentle neck stretches and work on the tail. You may not be sure where the lameness came from but, if you walk your horse, you may see a big improvement. Take a break or two during this procedure to determine if you are accomplishing anything, also to give the horse a chance to express how he is feeling. During these techniques, pay attention to the facial expressions of the horse, or have someone with you to report on how he is reacting and responding.

BACK PAIN

Back pain, if left untreated, can cause problems in other parts of the body, affecting gait and attitude. If you have checked for proper saddle fit, shoeing, and your own body condition and have found all these components in order, you may look to the back musculature or vertebral alignment for painful areas. Back pain is caused by injury, lack of sufficient turnout time, new training techniques, poor saddle fit, rider imbalance, stress (especially fear), overwork and internal organ problems. If you are not certain where the pain is, I suggest the following technique. It involves feeling energy without actually touching the horse and developing your senses in a new and exciting way for some of you. You will be seeing and feeling energy distortion without touching.

First, relax and center yourself. Stand about two feet away from your horse's back. With relaxed eyes, look at the area two or three inches above the spine. Beginning at the withers, scan along toward the tail. If all is well, you will not 'see' anything unusual. You may notice a distinctive difference between the area two or three inches above the body that is different from the area above and beyond. There should be a smoothness in this off-the-body manifestation of energy, with no open places, i.e. breaks in the aura. This indicates healthy, well-placed energy. In the area of pain or imbalance, you may perceive a 'disturbance in the force' to quote a line from *Star Wars*. This disturbance may look like waves of heat coming off the tar on the road on a hot day. It may look like smoke, or have a thickness to it that obscures your vision past the area into the distance. If you see anything of these manifestations or something similar, you may assume that it is a jitsu area, and the body is trying to disperse the excessive energy. This energy may be *jyaki*, the unbalanced, sick energy that sometimes occurs where there is a stagnation. Kyo energy looks like a hole in this smooth field, an opening in the aura that draws your eyes downward to the body and perhaps beyond the skin's surface. Make a mental note of everything you noticed.

Looking for kyo and jitsu without touching

Following the above scan, hold your relaxed hand above the horse's back. Keep your arm, elbow and shoulder, in addition to the rest of your body, extremely relaxed as you scan. Keep your hand at least two inches away, as holding it close in the hope of feeling more will distract you because you will feel the actual heat of the body, not the energy flow off the body. Pass your hand over the spine and Bladder Meridian on each side, moving it from the withers toward the tail. You may notice that you will not feel anything particularly interesting in the balanced areas. If energy is where it is supposed to be, it feels fine and does not catch your attention. The areas of distress will feel different. You may notice that in the areas where you previously saw some energetic discrepancy, you will feel something in your hand. You may feel an itchiness in your hand in areas of stagnation, where energy is stuck and unbalanced, especially if it has been so for a long time. This will help you when you do begin to touch the back, to know where to be especially gentle, not to disturb the horse, and lose his confidence in you. Spend time holding the kyo, or empty areas, until you feel some sensation in your hand, of circulation, vibration or any other manifestation of energy coming to the area. Masunaga said that if you work the kyo, the jitsu will take care of itself. I find this to be especially appropriate in the yin type horse who does not have too well defined jitsu. But in a yang horse, where there is a lot of jitsu, and perhaps not much kyo, it is necessary to work on the jitsu areas directly, even though it may be a bit uncomfortable for the horse at first. Go into the jitsu, tight areas, gradually but steadily building up pressure and speed. This will help disperse the energy that has been held, and the tension. Then slowly and patiently work the kyo.

Manifestations of jitsu

The jitsu areas may feel as if they are pushing your hand upward in the jitsu painful places. You may also feel something unusual in your palm, such as pressure, itching, tingling, or perhaps pain. The jitsu may feel warm or hot.

Manifestations of kyo

Kyo is more hidden and harder to find because of its subtlety. It is the depleted, underfunctioning condition that usually gives rise to the jitsu. The kyo areas feel as if they are drawing your hand downward to the surface of the body. Resist this feeling and complete the scan to the tail. The kyo, depleted and needing energy, feels empty. Nature hates a vacuum, hence the pulling feeling. The kyo may feel cool or cold.

It is the kyo and jitsu that need to be balanced. The energy from the jitsu needs to be dispersed, and hopefully dispersed into the depleted areas, rather than into another tight or painful place.

ARTHRITIS

If you have a horse without arthritis and have been doing regular shiatsu, you have a good chance of preventing its onset. Shiatsu keeps energy flowing and blocked energy is one cause of arthritis. Old injuries are the sites of arthritis. Regular shiatsu helps horses recover from injuries quickly and prevents them from being excessively traumatic. I believe that the non-habitual movement of the limbs during shiatsu gives the horse an additional 'vocabulary' of movement (this theory has been developed and discussed by Linda Tellington-Jones in her books), therefore, he may be able to immediately compensate with his body during an accident.

In dealing with old arthritic conditions, begin with very short sessions. It is too easy to aggravate the situation with an enthusiastic approach. Bringing too much circulation to a swollen area can be painful. Excessive manipulation of the limbs can irritate swollen joints. Avoid direct pressure where swelling is present. Where there is bone degeneration, little or no actual manipulation is advised.

When working on meridians that pass through swollen joints, avoid the area and follow instructions in the section on inflammation (*see* page 220). Your pressure should be slow and gentle. When the swelling subsides, you may begin small rotations in both directions. If one direction is easier and smoother, only rotate in that direction.

General shiatsu is advisable. Work on the entire body to promote healing and wellbeing. The Kidney Meridian relates to the bones and is a good one to work on during the session. The first session should be about twenty minutes long. Work on the Bladder and Kidney Meridians, and move anything that is not arthritic, even if it is only the tail or ears. Each joint has a relationship with every other joint, so promoting flexibility anywhere will have benefits for the less mobile parts. Work up to longer sessions slowly. It is possible that a very active session will promote flexibility immediately and miraculously, but the next day the horse may be more sore than ever. Work on Triple Heater Meridian for the lymphatic system and immune response. As the horse becomes accustomed to longer sessions that include gentle rotations and very minor stretches, take breaks during these sessions to walk a bit. The breaks will let your horse acclimatize to the new feelings of freedom within. In cases where the horse is too sensitive to receive hands-on work, acupuncture is advisable. This will get the energy moving and promote healing. Certain herbs and nutritional supplements may be helpful.

HEADACHES

Headaches may be caused by tension, both muscular and emotional. Allergies which cause blocked sinuses can create pressure, causing headaches. Jaw tension from grinding the teeth, or the wrong bit, can cause head pain, as can poor eyesight and fatigue. You may suspect your horse has a headache if he carries his head in a different position from the usual position, has a strained expression in his eyes, and is unresponsive to usual stimuli. Reluctance to wear a halter and especially a bridle are good indications of a headache.

There are many different types of headaches and understanding this will help you to treat them with shiatsu. For example, an injury that causes a misalignment or compression in the upper neck verte-brae can cause a headache. The techniques that release tension at the poll may be helpful in this case, as well as working on the Bladder Meridian. Unbalanced energy in the meridians may be the cause of headaches. Large Intestine Meridian imbalance may cause pain in the head in the location of this meridian. Low energy and top-of-the-head pain may be associated with Bladder Meridian. Any meridian that goes through the head area would be a good one to check if you suspect a headache. The way to check is to watch your horse move and look at which meridians are tight. Also, consider diet, environ-ment, and activities. Perhaps the bit is too severe for example.

Work on the suspected meridians and feel for tightness, blocked areas, excessive or depleted energy movement. Working on the meridian throughout the body will often help pain in a specific area. This is helpful to remember if there is an area you cannot touch because of injury. Working on the meridian elsewhere, as well as the other side, will move energy through the distressed area.

Generally, gentle shiatsu on the meridians of the neck will relax your horse enough to relieve the headache. If the headache persists, suspect some deeper problem. Give shiatsu to the three areas of the neck as described in the section on the neck (*see* pages 118–19), unless you know specifically which meridians to work on. Your technique should be slow and deliberate, gradually going in, holding, and grad-ually releasing each location, then making a smooth transition to the next one. If there is any resistance to any of the stretches, it could be because there is a vertebra out of alignment. Do not persist, just gently and patiently do as much as your horse will comfortably allow. Watch his eyes and expression as you work for clues as to exactly what is working, and what may be painful. Hold the points around the poll and ears with strong pressure, for as much time as it takes to feel energy unblocking. Release tension at the poll by doing the rocking side to side techniques, as well as tipping his nose toward his chest several times as you hold the points around the poll. Work around the eyes, perhaps several times, paying particular attention to the stretching outward of the outer corner of each eye. Work the cheek and inside the mouth several times to try to release the jaw tension that caused the headache or resulted from it. Work the forehead. Imagine what would feel good for you if you had such a headache.

> The first horse I ever worked with was suffering for months before I met him. He had reared and fallen over backwards, twisting his neck and lower spine. The neck injury resulted in a head tilt and headache. The second time I worked with him, I was intuitively moving his neck around when I heard a loud crack. I brought his head around to face forward and I saw the pain literally leave his eyes. The tilt was gone as his neck had adjusted itself; I just happened to be there at the time. There was a completely different look to his face. Because he was looking at me when the headache disappeared, he became bonded to me in a very unique way.

RUNNY EYES OR BLOCKED TEAR DUCTS

These problems are flip sides of the same coin, so the procedure for each is the same. Determine the cause of the problem if possible. Is there an allergic reaction to something in the environment, a foreign particle in the eye, a cold, or an injury? Give general shiatsu to the face, including ears, forehead, eyes, tear ducts, nose and mouth. Then work specifically on the Stomach Meridian in the face on both sides. Rework the tear ducts twice more, following through to and including the nostrils. Press points all around the forehead for a few minutes more. Work the mouth until your horse yawns.

FOUNDER (LAMINITIS)

Give general shiatsu without picking up any limbs. Standing on three legs will be too much of a strain for a horse with founder (laminitis). Move the energy in the legs with meridian work and jiggling. Work on Heart Constrictor and Triple Heater Meridians. Also work on Bladder and Kidney Meridians. Work on all the points around the coronary band (beginning and ending points of leg meridians front and back). After holding each point, work the meridian going upward if heat is felt in the feet. If the feet are cold, work downward on the leg meridians, holding the foot points at the end of each line. Do a dispersion technique of tapping the hooves with your knuckles. Do any technique that improves circulation, such as moving muscle in the hindquarters, and anything that feels pleasurable. Regular shiatsu is important during this extended period of enforced inactivity to keep circulation going and maintain a positive relationship in this time of physical and mental stress. A session each day is desirable, or perhaps two shorter sessions each day. Keep the horse relaxed since food is likely to be somewhat restricted.

> The summer of 1999 in northwestern New Jersey was a particularly dangerous one with respect to founder. We had a long dry spell, followed by a very rainy one. Little or no grass was replaced by rich lush grass almost overnight. The local vets reported many cases of founder, most of them fatal. My friend Cinnamon, was one of the victims. Already a fat little pony who everybody loves to give treats to because she is so cute, she was an accident waiting to happen. Because of some miscommunication, she was turned out on grass when she should not have been. The problem was seen to immediately, with everything the vet could do. I gave her regular shiatsu. She came through with flying colors, and is now back in light work and much happier. She has also lost weight and looks and feels wonderful.

INFLAMMATION

Inflammation is a natural mechanism for protection following trauma, but sometimes there can be excessive inflammation. Areas of inflammation are usually painful and cannot be touched directly. Ascertain exactly which meridians pass through the inflamed area. First, work the meridians on the uninjured limb. For example, if the left front leg is cut and swollen above the knee on the outside of the leg in the area of Triple Heater and Large Intestine, work those meridians in the right front leg. Then, on the injured leg, work with a very light and slow touch on these meridians, passing by the injury without touching it at all. You will be working above and below the swollen area. With a supporting hand on the foot, hold your other hand an inch or so away from the injury. Visualize healing taking place, or energy coming through your hand, or light. If the injury is radiating heat, think of your hand creating cooling energy, if the injury feels cold, project heat. Most of the time, inflammation creates heat. Do general shiatsu on the Bladder Meridian. Keep all the feet on the ground. Give shiatsu each day during healing. Try to keep your horse relaxed while healing energy does its work.

COLDS

Refer also to the section on runny eyes and blocked tear ducts on page 219. Colds come when the immune system is low. When the first line of defense, the Lung Meridian, is out of balance, the body can 'catch' a cold. The Lung Meridian governs resistance to external intrusions, such as airborne and surface germs and irritants. Triple

Heater Meridian helps support the function of the lymphatic system. Both these meridians are beneficial for helping move the cold out of the body. Concentrate on the beginning and ending points of these meridians. Also work on Kidney Meridian for vitality, and Liver Meridian for detoxification. It is important for the horse to get adequate rest so the body's energy can build up. Time off is advisable. Even if you get immediate results and the cold seems much better, give the horse a rest. Work on your horse every day until the cold's symptoms diminish, then work every second day. Do a lot of grooming to stimulate the skin because it relates to the lungs and is an organ of detoxification. Do a once-a-week session after the symptoms have completely disappeared to support the immune system and prevent another cold from taking hold. Determine if the cold is yin or yang in nature and work accordingly. A yin cold involves a lot of running clear mucus, a yang cold produces thick mucus that has a greenish color. Work slowly and with lots of holding for a yin cold, work more quickly and with strong pressure for a yang cold. Unfortunately for the horse, the symptoms may be exacerbated as a result of treatment because they are coming out faster than they would without treatment. The good news is that the duration of the cold will be greatly shortened. There are herbal remedies and homeopathic remedies that are helpful.

COLIC

These techniques should be employed immediately after calling your vet. The points at the very tip of each ear are the ones to concentrate on when your horse shows the first sign of colic. If you have been working regularly on your horse, he will have no objection to work on the ears. Walk your fingers alternately up the ear, with your thumbs on the inside and your four fingertips on the outside. When you reach the tip, gently press and squeeze between your thumb and index finger. Your supporting hand should be back at the base of the ear, holding the head gently in ear rotation position. Hold the tip steadily for about thirty seconds, release briefly, hold for thirty seconds and continue in this manner until you have worked on the tip point for a few minutes. Proceed to the other ear and work the same way. If your horse begins to lower his head and relax, proceed to the points on the Bladder Meridian just before the hindquarters. The first point to hold is at the junction of the thoracic and lumbar vertebrae, and the second is centered above the tuber coxae. Hold these points simultaneously for about a minute on each side. Then listen for gut sounds. Go back to the ears and work on them using all the ear techniques, concentrating on the tip points each time you get there.

Stretch the hind legs forward and backward several times, holding each stretch position for at least ten seconds for maximum release. Do percussion on the large muscles of the hindquarters. Work on Stomach, Large Intestine and Small Intestine Meridians. Even if you hear normal gut sounds and see your horse relax long before you have completed all the techniques, continue to do them all, walking the horse often.

POSTSURGICAL TECHNIQUES

If your horse has gone away to have surgery and you are permitted to visit during the recovery period, it is crucial to touch him as much as possible. This touching can be in the form of stroking, simply holding, or whatever seems appropriate. Talk to him, sing to him, and keep him in the conscious world. Know when he needs a break to sleep, since rest is a great healer. He will do better while away from home if you are allowed contact. Consult the vet about giving shiatsu. Avoid any technique that requires the horse to stand on three legs.

You may work gently on the Liver Meridian to help the body detoxify from anesthesia, and support the detoxification process during recovery. Work on Kidney Meridian to support the filtration of fluids, as well as Bladder Meridian. Work on Stomach Meridian to encourage appetite for food and appetite for life. Work on Lung Meridian for resistance to external intrusions as the immune system may be a bit compromised at this time. Stimulate his skin, which is a mirror of the lungs, and is the largest organ in the body, according to traditional Chinese medicine. Let him hear you breathing deeply. This may remind him to breathe too, and will help release toxins and keep both of you healthy. These meridians may be incorporated into a more complete session after your horse has returned home. Make him as comfortable as possible and baby him a lot. Try some fresh carrot juice, for both of you.

SHOCK AND TRAUMA

Reassure your horse with your voice and hands, even if you are not sure he is aware of you at all. Breathe deeply and audibly to encourage your horse to do the same. This deep even breathing into your lower abdomen will help keep you centered along with your horse. Do the all-over stroking technique with a strong firm touch. Keep your hands firmly on your horse as a light pressure may not be felt at this time, or be annoying. Work on Small Intestine Meridian to support balance, as this is the first meridian to register shock. Use Governing Vessel 26 for shock and loss of consciousness. It is located on the midline between the lowest portion of the nostrils. Hold this point with firm deep pressure for thirty seconds for at least three minutes. Keep talking to your horse and reassuring him, even after things return to normal. The memory of this ordeal will cause your horse to react strongly to other situations for awhile, so be patient and give regular gentle shiatsu for at least two months after the trauma. There are herbs and Bach Flower Remedies for shock that will help.

TYING UP (AZOTURIA)

Sooth and calm your horse with your voice and hands.
Concentrate on working the Bladder Meridian thoroughly for its

relationship with azoturia and impetus. Work strongly, deeply and quickly at first, as this is a jitsu condition, then work slowly on the points of the meridian, on each side, beginning just behind the withers and ending with rotation of the vertebrae of the tail. Work the meridian again, and finish at the ending points in the feet, holding each point for about thirty seconds, and finish with a tail stretch. Gently jiggle the neck and work on Bladder Meridian in the neck. Work straight through to the last points on the foot on each side, then do the side to side stretches of the tail, the lifting arc, vertebrae rotations, and stretch. During the stretch hold for five seconds, then release a bit, stretch again for ten seconds, release a bit and stretch for thirty seconds. Work on Gall Bladder and Liver Meridians to help with detoxification. Jiggle the legs without lifting them. Use percussion on the hindquarters with cupped hands. During this procedure, if your horse begins to move a bit, you may attempt to walk him briefly, then finish your shiatsu.

> In my early years as a practitioner I was working as a volunteer at the US Equestrian Team three-day event and had never heard of tying up at the time. I was paged to the stall of a horse with this particular problem. It had happened before and he was looking miserable and frightened (note that the emotion associated with the Bladder Meridian is fear). The problem was briefly explained to me so I did what seemed like a logical sequence of work on the Bladder Meridian, then working Gall Bladder and Liver Meridians for their muscle, tendon, and ligament relationship and for detoxification. I could feel that there was a jitsu condition throughout the back, so I worked deeply and quickly at first, then slowed to work deeply and deliberately. As the muscles began to ease and the horse's head began to lower, I realized that he was not only relaxing, but was also stretching his own Bladder Meridian. I tried to walk him out then and he looked frightened again. I knew this was due to old patterns and ideas, so I coaxed him and reassured him with my voice (I can be very seductive when sweet-talking a horse) and he followed me right out of the stall. His owner was amazed, as previously only drugs could ease this situation. He eagerly learned some techniques to help his horse. I told him that prevention could help and that he should work regularly on his horse to prevent the problem from ever occurring again.

NAVICULAR

Work the entire body to promote circulation and the sense of wholeness. This is especially important to the horse who has been in work and is now suddenly without any job but standing around trying to recover from a painful condition. Full body shiatsu will release natural painkillers in the horse's body. The typical navicular/founder stance is one of stiffness throughout the body, and general shiatsu will promote healing and flexibility. If your horse suddenly feels pain free and exuberant do not let him run too much as he will be sore later. Concentrate on the front of the horse to begin with. Work the shoulder and foreleg to bring circulation to the feet. Heart Constrictor Meridian, with its relationship to the veins and arteries, will help bring circulation to the feet. Triple Heater Meridian will help regulate body temperature and keep excessive heat out of the feet. Stay several seconds on the terminal point of the Heart Constrictor Meridian. It is between the bulbs of the front heels in a hollow. Work on the points in the front feet without lifting the legs. Using your knuckles or the end of a riding crop, knock on the hooves, all around, to promote circulation. Work the Bladder Merdian and use the stretching techniques on the actual meridian (*see* page 71). Work the back and hindquarters to bring the horse's attention and awareness here and away from the painful shoulders, feet and legs. If pain is present in the front legs when working, work very gently and at medium speed on the meridians. If there is heat in the feet and legs, visualize the painful energy leaving the leg and going down and outward, dispersing itself. Work on the Liver Meridian to help disperse toxins in the body accumulated during inactivity.

MOUTHINESS

Horses interact with the world around them with all their senses, and especially their mouths. As you give shiatsu, your horse may feel like reciprocating with grooming and nibbling. This is cute but distracting and may even be dangerous, since the shiatsu is releasing blocked energy and the nuzzling could quickly turn into nipping. I discourage these attentions while I am working as I need to concentrate on what I am feeling, and so should the horse on whom I am working. Save the snuggling and licking until after the session. Use all the techniques for the mouth, gums and cheeks (*see* pages 136–42) to release tension in the mouth, since mouthiness is often an expression of tension or pain (check the inside of the cheeks for lesions caused by sharp teeth).

When working on an orally fixated horse, I do the mouth and cheek work first. This gives the horse something to think about, and he will spend a long time chewing and licking, mulling over the sensations from the work there.

When working on one particularly mouthy fellow who thought I must be delicious, I worked on his mouth early in the session. Every time he tried to bite me, the yawn reflex took over each time he began to open his mouth. It was funny how he could not close his mouth anywhere near me during the entire session.

'HOPELESS' CASES

Many students have come to me in frustration because they have been asked to work on a severely abused and frightened horse on whom they have tried everything but cannot get the horse to relax and accept treatment. Some are fearful of attempting to work with horses who display signs of aggression. Others are told a horse is a lost cause. I recommend Henry Blake's books *Talking with Horses, Horse Sense, Thinking with Horses* (Souvenir Press) for advice on dealing with severe behavior problems before trying to give shiatsu. Eventually, you may be able to touch the horse somewhere where your touch will be accepted. Incorporate shiatsu into the way you touch, even if it is only a small area. Gradually expand this area as you become more trusted. Always leave him wanting a bit more so you are greeted enthusiastically and receptively the next time. Be patient, never rush. This horse is an investment in time, so if you feel you do not have the time for an ongoing project, find someone who does. Never let your guard down, even when the horse seems relaxed. Something outside the stall could trigger a flight response that the horse is not in control of. Unpleasant memories get very stuck and cause very quick actions.

One of my students was attending a Monty Roberts clinic where there was a horse who was very ill, in pain and dangerous. My student, a very petite young woman, had recently attended my Level 1 course. She felt so sorry for this poor creature she asked permission to try shiatsu to make him more comfortable. She was reluctantly given permission but only if she wore protective clothing, including a helmet. She began by kneeling in the corner of the stall. This 'dangerous' horse went quietly over to investigate. She slowly arose and gently and cautiously began the session. The results were so remarkable and surprising for everyone (though not my student) that Mr. Roberts was called over to see the change.

PAIN

Expressions of pain

Horses are good communicators, especially regarding their own needs. While hunger may be expressed in obvious ways, pain, in some stoic types, may be more difficult to detect. During any session of shiatsu or any other form of bodywork therapy, keep keenly aware of your horse's reactions. The narrowing of an eye, tilt of an ear or lowering of the head with the rearward tilt of an ear, are some indications you have touched something sensitive. Bared teeth and lifted legs are usually a last resort in normally well-adjusted horses dealing with some physical stress. There are horses, with a history of abuse, who will either walk away from you as soon as you contact a sore area or become aggressive. Know the horse and his history before attempting shiatsu. Your visual observation techniques will help you to stay safe and be effective.

Painful points

If a point is chronically painful, check the meridian line on which it is located. Check the rest of the meridian for sensitivity. If there are other areas of distress on the particular meridian that do not diminish with time and shiatsu, you may consider that there is an imbalance or some distress in the organ related to the meridian. Also, consider the emotional qualities associated with the particular meridian.

Work on the meridian in front of and past the painful point, and the entire meridian on the other side of the body. Check the point again. If it is still sensitive, hold your supporting hand over the point with no pressure and work as much of the meridian as you can reach with fairly deep pressure. Check the point again. If it is still sensitive and on a limb, you may stretch the meridian in an attempt to release this blocked energy. You may also work on the paired meridian on both sides. If the area is on the back, walk your horse for a few minutes after working on the back then feel again. If it is still sensitive, wait until a day has passed as energy sometimes takes a day or two to respond to treatment. If it is still sensitive after a few days, perhaps try some herbal remedies for general wellbeing. Do not overstimulate the area by overworking it. You may take a few days break from treatment and try again.

Dealing with severe pain and new injuries

The emotional trauma associated with the pain of a fresh injury may very well preclude you from working with shiatsu immediately. If the trauma includes swelling, it may be advisable to wait for one day before doing shiatsu, although having your hands reassuringly supporting your horse is important during this time. Let the body begin its healing process as you help with the appropriate first-aid techniques.

A traumatized area is overly stimulated by the bodily response and should not be touched immediately. This is a case of jitsu protecting kyo, or jitsu hiding kyo. When the pain has settled down a bit, use tonification techniques, working distally until energy begins moving through the meridian along which the injury has occurred. You may hold your hand over the injured area without touching, just radiating healing energy as you touch other areas. You may use visualization techniques, such as the pain lifting and rising out of your horse. If the pain could have a color, what would it be? Imagine that color rising out.

When you do touch the injured place eventually, do so with your entire palm rather than thumb or fingertips. The touch should be like that of a butterfly, landing and rising gently. Trust your instincts as to how long to stay, and when to begin to increase your pressure. Pay close attention to your horse's response and keep him in a trusting and relaxed attitude. Any squeamishness or hesitancy from you will be felt by your horse, so only touch when you also feel confident. Use your other hand in a way that will distract your horse from the injured site. For example, scratch or tap an area nearby simultaneously.

Work along the meridian line going to and from the injury. Your supporting hand could be near the injured place as a monitor of how much energy you actually feel moving. Work on the same meridian completely on the other side of the body which will have a positive effect on the injured side. This is called the 'see-saw phenomena'.

When the swelling subsides, your touch will be more easily accepted on the injured area. As your horse heals and the injury no longer poses a problem, avoid calling attention to it by repeatedly touching it or poking it as you show people where the injury was. This will only create a lasting memory and possible enduring psychological and physical pain.

BORED HORSES

Most habits we find annoying in horses are the result of too much time when they are not occupied or stimulated, especially mentally. Hours confined in the stall away from companions will, most assuredly, cause the horse to chew his surroundings, wind suck, weave etc. Some horses turn inward mentally and become antisocial. Boring and repetitive work under saddle can cause a bright horse to become dull and uninterested in the activities at hand. Horses need variety, mental and physical stimulation, and it is the owner's responsibility to provide it.

Learn how to teach your horse some fun and *safe* tricks. Provide toys for him to play with such as large balls to kick around or something hanging from his stall he can knock about. He will eventually become bored with these things so use your creativity to find other interesting pastimes for him. I have seen many horses benefit from the work Pat Parelli teaches. His training techniques will increase your knowledge and patience tremendously and help your horse to develop mentally. It will increase the bond between you; if you are bored with life, your horse will pick up on it. Inspire each other. Play. Dance. Celebrate life!

Getting the Horse Accustomed to Treatment

Your horse needs to learn how to receive a treatment, just as you must learn the fine nuances of giving one. Gear your work to the personality and energy type of the horse. Understanding your horse in all facets of his bodymindspirit will contribute to your successful relationship with each other, letting your horse know you will keep the positive energy running both ways.

When you begin to work with a horse not accustomed to bodywork of any sort, keep your session short and simple. For example, following the beginning technique of all-over stroking, work on the Bladder Meridian on the back, rotate the legs, do a bit of jiggling, and close the session with all-over stroking again. Reassure him throughout the session that he is doing a great job as recipient. The next time, repeat this procedure and add some work on leg meridians and perhaps a little neck work. Gradually work up to a full hour. Of course, some horses will be happy to let you do everything you can think of the first time they receive a session. It seems as if they have been waiting all their lives for shiatsu, and they act as if it is the most perfect thing ever. There will be times when a horse just does not wish to be worked on, and persisting may result in you getting nipped, or reluctance to receive treatment another time. Do not persist just because you have set aside this time. Work within the needs and desires of the horse but consider that he may be so sore that everything hurts. In this case it may be better to wait until tomorrow. Perhaps only work on the ears and feet, without lifting the leg.

ATMOSPHERE

The atmosphere for healing is relatively simple to create. Of course, the atmosphere must start within the practitioner as well as the surrounding area, which will be discussed later. Wherever you work, both of you should feel safe, comfortable and relaxed. Try to work during a time well away from feeding time and when the area is quiet. If there are disruptive horses in the area, work somewhere else. You may notice after the session that all the horses in the area have become relaxed along with your horse. Let people in the area know you are giving a session so that noise can be kept to a minimum. If someone begins asking you questions about what you are doing, tell them you must concentrate while you work and will be happy to answer their queries after you have finished. If working in the stall, it should be clean and large enough to allow for leg stretches.

Remove food, but keep the water bucket accessible. On rare occasions I will allow a horse to munch hay while I work if he is a particularly nervous or mouthy horse, or physically very sensitive. If you choose to play music, it should be soft and peaceful. I prefer to work without a halter inside the stall but sometimes it is safer for the horse to wear one. Occasionally I may tie the horse in the stall if he continues to wander around. Sometimes I have the owner with me holding the horse on a lead rope. If this is the case, ask the owner to try not to touch or fuss with the horse while you are working. I give them the job of reporting all the facial expressions as I work. From time to time, I work with a horse in cross ties. This is helpful if the stall is small or if the footing is too deep for me to be balanced. If working outside the stall, it is preferable to have someone hold the horse. Some horses concentrate better if the owner is not present at all. There are some horses I can work on in the barn aisle without having to tie them up; they would not dream of wandering away while I work on them. Above all, you and the horse need to be safe, so check any area in which you are working for obstacles. If working in the aisle, make sure there are no ropes on the floor, or slippery areas nearby. Working outside is lovely if there are no other horses in the area. Horses are curious and can be distracting and disruptive to both of you if they gather round while you are trying to work.

TRUSTING YOUR INSTINCTS

Your intuition is your greatest tool. Coupled with education, it is invaluable. The expanded awareness of your work when you trust that wise voice inside you will guide you truthfully and successfully.

It may be difficult at first to trust your instincts but, like a muscle that grows stronger with proper work, your instincts will become stronger and you will become wiser as you exercise your intuition.

Unfortunately, most of us are not encouraged to trust this innate ability and we lose access to it, even though it is always there. To get back to this natural state of insight (inner sight), we must quiet our minds and listen. Listen to the quiet and peace within. Allow yourself to be in an expanded state of consciousness, limitless. This limitlessness is a state of awareness in which you can feel at one with the universe. If you are able to be in this open state of being, your intuition will flow. Listen and flow with the answers. Let go of the sometimes troublesome intellect and ego, and trust. Gently let go of any doubts that may form. They will keep you from hearing the entire message. Be joyous in the knowledge that you are under-standing yourself and becoming one with the universe.

Yin and Yang Horse Types and Understanding Them

Most horses (as well as people and other developed creatures) are, ideally, a combination of yin and yang qualities. Understanding your horse from an energetic viewpoint will foster harmony, understanding and success in your relationship. Understanding yourself also in this context will help you to choose the right horse for your temperament. A balanced individual is able to express a full range of emotions. However, these reactions need to be expressed at appropriate times. For example, many of us do not approve of the expression of anger. We repress it in our horses and ourselves. Anger is a natural emotion and holding it back when it would be appropriate to express it is unhealthy and perhaps dangerous. It is still inside and may be building, only to come out at inappropriate times. Let the energy flow!

THE YIN HORSE

In general, the yin horse is delicate physically and emotionally. His bones may be long, slender and refined. His coat is soft and silky and his features aristocratic in an ethereal way. During a crisis, he may fall apart emotionally and take ages to recover. He is like the Southern belle who gets the vapors and goes into a swoon or a tizzy at the least surprise. He may take a long time to recover from illness. He may have trouble expressing himself as everything gets held inside until he becomes either physically ill, or has some sort of emotional breakdown. His physical injuries may come from overusing muscles that do not have the healthy contraction needed to keep them from overstretching and tearing. His ligaments and tendons may get injured easily. A typical example of the yin horse is the Thoroughbred racehorse, all nervous energy, thin and fragile.

The yin horse may be a finicky eater and a poor keeper, or may be obsessed with food and bolt it down without tasting it. If this is the case, the horse may still be thin even though he is eating a lot of food because the nutrients are not being absorbed thoroughly since the digestive process begins in the mouth with saliva breaking down the components of food.

The horse with a yin personality tends to be an overthinker and a worrier. You can see him weighing all the possibilities. Everything has the potential to upset him; there are ghosts everywhere. He remembers every unpleasant thing that ever happened to him without being able to let go and relax. He takes ages to adjust to new surroundings, unless his owner is extra careful to prepare him for the change.

THE YANG HORSE

A yang horse is a sturdier type both physically and emotionally. He has heavy bones, solid muscle structure, which may be prone to spasms, and a disposition that allows him to cruise through life in an accepting and mellow way. His coat is probably less refined than that of the yin horse. He usually recovers quickly from illness, however, his illnesses may be quite severe, sometimes with a heartbreaking outcome. Clydesdales, Percherons and other breeds of heavy horses and ponies are examples of yang types. A horse with a yang personality is usually a solid citizen and a safe ride. He will take good care of you and your family, indeed, may be a member of your family. Although this horse will remember everything from the past, he will not dwell on it and let it influence the present. The flip side of this aspect is the stoic type who holds everything inside and does not allow himself to be expressive. This is an extremely patient and forgiving creature. The yang horse may be stubborn and difficult to convince at times. It is easy to assume that the big, strong, easy-going yang type does not have a great deal of sensitivity but he may be delicate in his inner self even though he presents a stoic facade.

There are, however, combinations to consider. You may have a physically yang horse who is mentally a yin type, or a physically yin horse who is emotionally yang. These characteristics should be kept in mind when approaching him to give shiatsu, and should also be taken into account with all his other activities.

WORKING ON A YIN HORSE

A yin type horse needs more delicate and refined work, with great sensitivity to every subtle reaction during the session. This horse may become overly stimulated by the energy released during your work, and lose his attention span. Begin the session in a way that mimics the energy of the horse. For example, if the horse is busy and fussy, begin with fairly fast work and vary your technique to get and keep the horse's attention. When the horse becomes more focussed, begin to slow your work down a bit. You will be gradually getting him to relax as you work more and more slowly to the end. Even if you have a very spaced-out horse for awhile, it is beneficial to induce such a deep state of relaxation in a nervous horse. Keep this horse in his stall after the session so he does not fall over his own feet. It may be advisable to take a break or two to walk him in-hand, to get him gradually accustomed to the new sensations in his body. Even if he has no physical problems, give him the rest of the day off the first time you give him a really relaxing full session. The effects of shiatsu are cumulative, so your nervous horse will generally become much mellower with regular sessions.

The yin horse may do well with shorter sessions at first so as not to overload his senses, or risk losing his attention. You may not need to hold the points for very long as the quick-moving energy of the yin horse, if he is a nervous type, responds almost immediately. When doing any stretches, do not hold them for too long because the physically yin horse may not contract easily after prolonged stretching; also, do not overstretch! Be certain that everyone in the area knows that you need a quiet atmosphere in which to work, for this horse may easily be startled. If the highly strung yin horse falls asleep, consider it a huge compliment!

WORKING ON A YANG HORSE

This horse will be extremely forgiving of even your clumsiest and inexperienced efforts. He accepts shiatsu like it is no big deal, at first. He grooms you as you work on him because he is so accommodating, or else he just goes to sleep and practically falls over on you while you are holding up one of his legs. You may need to get his energy moving a bit before you begin the session or else you will not be able to feel his energy moving at all. Perhaps you should take him for a walk on a lead line, and trot him a little as well. Show him some area of his environment he has not seen before, sing him a song or dance for him. When he is a bit more switched on, begin your session. The all-over stroking could be done quickly to spark him up, talk or sing to him a bit as you work. After you really have his attention, begin to fine-tune your work to teach him the delicate as well as the strong nuances of energy moving throughout his body. Try to keep him from falling asleep during the actual session. Percussion techniques may stimulate his interest and energy. Jiggles will help those tight muscles to loosen. Prolonged stretches will give his muscles the time they need to relax and release. You can give him strong and solid pressure.

Following a treatment, or a series of treatments, a horse may change his mind about something. For example, I taught some courses at a facility that catered to disabled riders. Their horses were some of the practice horses for my students. The manager put cards on each stable door giving a brief description of each horse. One of the disabled riders' horses, a huge black heavy horse named Percy, I was told did not like to jump. He would walk over jumps no matter how the rider tried to get him to do otherwise. After a few days as one of our shiatsu guinea pigs, the manager told me that Percy had uncharacteristically trotted up to a jump and jumped right over without any unusual prompting by the rider. The young man riding him was ecstatic and shocked, and did not fall off. Percy had changed his mind!

Please note that a yang horse can suffer from a yin type ailment, and a yin type horse can suffer from a yang type ailment, which will be mentioned later.

PAIRING HORSE AND RIDER ACCORDING TO TYPE

When buying a horse, most people make a choice which is based on many things: age, breed, type of work, training level, prior accomplishments, personality, etc. I have heard many stories about people who went to look at a horse and bought it without knowing too much about it at all. They state that it was love at first sight, or that the horse chose them.

I have seen some combinations of horse and owner that I could not understand as they seemed so blatantly unsuited to each other. The harmonious combination of temperaments between horse and person is ideal of course and, with guidance, many great partnerships are formed.

Knowing whether you are a yin or yang type person may help you to choose the perfect horse for you. Choosing a horse with some similar personality traits to those you have can avoid too many problems later. If you are a calm patient type of person without prize-winning ambitions and choose a horse needing slow handling because of prior abuse and injuries, you have a good chance of gradually helping the horse become whole again. You would need to be open-minded and willing to try anything and everything until you hit upon just the right thing, or combination of therapies, to help this horse. A young inexperienced and nervous rider would only be asking for trouble with this type of horse. A yang type person who is very outgoing, strong, easygoing and takes charge, may not do well with a temperamental horse who is highly strung, as they perhaps would not be able to understand the horse's flightiness, or worse, not have the patience to persevere with him. A yin, delicate person, shy, perhaps introverted, may have trouble handling a big yang, fearless horse, who takes charge of all situations. Even so, this type of horse would take care of this person and perhaps be a positive influence, causing the person to become more self-assured and outgoing.

One of my students bought a 'difficult' horse for very little money, and I can understand why. At first glance, he looked beautiful and spirited but upon closer examination he revealed many physical and emotional problems. His new owner was working with him slowly to gain his trust. He would only accept his owner in his stall with him and no one else. She stated that after several months he still was not able to accept or give affection, but at least he was no longer aggressive. She brought him to a Level 1 course. During these courses, students practice in pairs inside the stall, with one person holding the horse while the other one practices. The horse holder's job is to report facial expressions to the person practicing to gauge the response to each technique, and to protect them from getting nibbled. This owner chose as her partner one of the older women in the class, another very patient and sweet horse person. From the quiet way she entered the stall with the owner, the horse made no objection. He resisted either of them working on him until he realized that shiatsu was not so bad. He began to relax and allowed the new person to practice when his owner had finished. He was still a bit defensive but made no real objections. Each time I looked in on them to give praise and suggestions, I observed the horse's head getting lower and lower. By the end of the first day of practice, he was soft and sleepy. On the morning of the second day he was asking for affection and shiatsu, and nuzzling his owner, resting his forehead on her chest while she touched his ears (something she had not been able to do for the entire time she had him), and giving her kisses. She was so moved and happy, as was I. Having gained his trust, she was able to begin to make him more comfortable. He moved with much more fluidity at the end of the course.

Possible Session Procedures

Try to make all your sessions interesting as well as effective. Avoid doing the same procedure over and over again but, initially, it may be advantageous to have a set routine until you are sure enough of yourself to try some variations. Having a routine in mind, with respect to the needs of the horse of course, will help you avoid worrying about what to do next, until you become proficient enough to do your session based entirely on the needs of the horse. Ohashi always tells his students 'when in doubt, rotate'; good advice for horse work as well as people work.

GENERAL SESSIONS

A good general session might consist of:

- All-over stroking
- Bladder Meridian on the back
- Shoulder (front leg) jiggle and rotation, each leg
- Front foot rotation and foot flop followed by stretching each leg
- One or two meridians on the front legs
- Hindquarters palming, leg rotation, resting on toe jiggle, other leg
- Hind leg stretches
- One or two meridians
- Tail work
- Neck and face work
- All-over stroking

OR

- All-over stroking
- Bladder Meridian on the back
- Neck work on both sides
- Shoulder (front leg) jiggle and shoulder work on both sides
- Rocking knee lift and full stretch
- Rear leg jiggle in each direction, rotations and stretches on both legs
- Tail work
- Face work
- All-over stroking

OR

- All-over stroking
- Three meridians in the neck
- Two or three meridians in the front legs
- Shoulder meridians
- Bladder Meridian continuing to Bladder Meridian in rear legs
- One or two more rear leg meridians
- All legs rotated and stretched (optional)
- Tail work
- Two simple neck stretches
- Face work
- All-over stroking

PRERIDE TREATMENT

- All-over stroking
- Palming the Bladder Meridian from withers to tail
- Incremental movement of the neck, followed by neck side stretch
- Rotations of front feet, shoulders, and leg stretches
- Rotation of the back feet and legs with stretches
- Stretching the tail
- Work inside the mouth
- All-over stroking

POSTRIDE TREATMENT

- All-over stroking
- Palming the back and deep work with palms all over the hind-quarters
- Rear leg jiggles
- Shoulder (front leg) jiggles
- Neck jiggle and stretch
- Ears
- Cheeks
- All-over stroking

The possibilities and combinations of techniques are endless. Just consider the special needs of the horse you are working on, not only generally, but also specifically in his present condition, in the present moment.

Also consider your condition. If you are tired or have an injury, you may wish to avoid strenuous movement such as rotations and big stretches. Meridian work alone can be effective in promoting flexibility in your horse. You may find though, that after you work on your horse you feel better, regardless of how you felt when you began the session.

Trust your instincts regarding your capabilities. Listen to that wise inner voice. You may find that if you do not feel well, your sensitive horse will pick up on the fact, and perhaps show reluctance to receive a treatment.

In 1985 I was working fairly regularly with a huge, sweet warm-blood. He was always ready for shiatsu. He impressed me with his intelligence and sensitivity, and so I was never reluctant to drive the two and a half hours to see him. I had just moved from my New York City apartment into a house in the country and on the morning of the day I was to see him I had to saw a low limb off one of my trees. The job gave me an instant sore shoulder and back as I was not accustomed to this type of labor. That afternoon at the barn (a beautiful structure built in the round, like an old Shaker barn, owned by Calvin Klein), my old friend would not let me lift his back legs. Anything else was fine. I had walked him and knew he was not sore in the legs or hindquarters. I kept trying to lift a leg, which irritated my injury, but after driving all that way I was determined to give him the full extent of my techniques. I finally stood by his beautiful head and asked him silently why he was resisting, and the answer came back, 'you have pain and I don't'. That touched me deeply. I thanked him for his consideration and continued the session without trying to pick up his back legs. I was developing my listening skills.

There was another horse at that location who gave me an 'earful'. She was an Arabian driving horse. Her owners, a couple who loved her very much and thought they understood her completely, called her 'Mother'. They asked me to see her because her gait had become uneven and the vet could not find anything wrong with her. I watched her move and saw a neck problem, and took her to her stall to begin the session. I knelt and asked her silently to share anything she wanted to with me. Suddenly, I was overwhelmed by a feeling of sadness and in my mind's eye I saw a foal. I tried to interpret this information. Perhaps she had had a foal that died. No, that did not feel like an answer. Then it hit me loud and clear: she was seeing a foal somewhere everyday and was aching to have one herself. I was so overwhelmed by this information that I excused myself from her for a moment and looked for her owners. I asked, 'Is there a mare and foal here that she sees every day?' I was told a mare had recently given birth in the stall next to hers and was turned out with the baby in a paddock where their mare could just see them from a distance when she was turned out. Now, imagine a stranger about to tell you something about the horse you think you understand so well, I had to be careful not to offend them. I explained my impressions and told them she wanted very much to have a foal. They said she had been bred, but not for years, and they had no immediate plans to breed her as she was in regular competition. I asked them to arrange for her to be turned out in the same pasture or an adjoining one so that she could have contact with the new foal. I then went back to her and finished the session. My work was successful and after the session she was moving perfectly again. I was learning how to listen and interpret.

Learning to Listen

This is a skill that must be practiced constantly. My own listening skills are still being developed and refined. Since I travel to different countries to teach, it is especially important when trying to communicate with someone for whom English is a second language, even if fluent. Even in Great Britain, I find the style of dialogue so different from America that I must really concentrate and hear, as well as listen. From state to state in the US, communication styles are varied as well. When teaching, there may be a tremendous diversity of nationalities in my students. I must communicate with them effectively, taking nothing for granted.

Animal communicators are plentiful these days and many people get help from them. It is sometimes not easy to be objective when your own love and worry are clouding your hearing. These people have a variety of ways in which they work. Each has found the way in which they clearly receive information. They can all teach us something but each one of us needs to find our own unique style of sending and receiving information. I have found that if I empty my mind (not hard to do) and wait patiently while breathing deeply into my center, often information comes clearly. Sometimes I get pictures in my mind or perhaps my imagination. Sometimes a word or phrase comes in a whisper so soft I can barely hear it. But if my mind is uncluttered and quiet, I can hear the whisper quite clearly. One of the early books that influenced me was *Kinship With All Life* by J. Allen Boone (Harper Collins). In this book, Mr. Boone describes how he regarded all beings as an expression of the infinite mind of God. He also tried to communicate not as a higher being to a lower being, but as an equal.

Horses speak to us in many ways. The easiest and most obvious way is through body language. The common facial language expressions are placing the ears forward, sideways or back, holding their mouths tight with set jaws, various eye expressions and movement of the nostrils. The larger movements are shying, running away, rearing and refusing to move by planting all four feet. Horses are great communicators.

In the December 1999 issue of *The Whole Horse Journal*, Diana Thompson speaks about how labeling hinders listening. In the horse industry there is an equestrian slang of words and expressions describing behavior in horses that is problematic to interaction with people and their demands. Each riding style has its phrases. The ones I hear in Great Britain are particularly colorful. Diana says, 'the use of these words interferes with the two-way communication which is crucial to a good human-horse partnership. Once we label the horse's actions with one of these terms, we tend to stop listening. We don't pause to figure out why the horse is acting a certain way. We observe the action, label it, and then, as if the action never occurred, continue to demand what we want'.

Look for your horse's problem and listen to his 'speech'. Reluctance to perform can usually be analyzed and corrected, especially in the early stages. Horses are not intractable or disobedient for the fun of it. They may be confused by unclear cues from the rider, or fearful. They may not be educated well enough to understand what you want. They may also be unfit and unable to perform as you would wish. Fearfulness is a huge cause of communication problems; when fear kicks in, communication is practically impossible.

If your horse is displaying any actions that can be 'labeled', take a few minutes to ask why he is behaving in this way. Check to see if your cues are clear and your communication is a two-way street. Give shiatsu to determine if there is pain anywhere. Check for proper saddle fit, mouth pain and sore feet. Did something in his environment disturb your horse recently, and has sleep been disturbed as a result?

I have a friend, Nancy Orlen Weber, who says there is a constant stream of information, past and present, that is always flowing by, and all we need to learn to do is tap into it. Nancy says, 'Know that within every living being there is a divine presence operating the life force. This continuous flow of energy ignites the individual mind with an infinite source of wisdom, knowledge and the ability to translate the information from any other species. Approach each sentient being with a consciously open heart and know that the universal stream of life is shared between you and the other being. Imagine your personal mind is one layer of circuits within an overlapping universal circuitry that interacts with your personal mind. This universal circuitry flows throughout the universe, shared by all of life. Trusting the processing between personal and universal flow allows for the immediate translation of images, thoughts, feelings and physiology of a horse, a dog, a cat, a fly, or any other brethren sharing this incredible planet.'

Taking Breaks

When first acclimatizing your horse to full body shiatsu sessions, it may become necessary to take a break or two during the course of the actual treatment. The short break allows the horse time to relax and feel the sensations and reactions of healing. It is a time for your horse to relax and focus inward, in a quiet and healing atmosphere. A break can also give you time to recenter yourself and take a rest during an intense session.

Some horses have a short attention span and, if this is the case, I would rather stop before the horse loses concentration, have a change of scenery, then go back to work. Some horses become so relaxed and spaced-out during shiatsu, they switch off completely. Unless the horse has been in so much pain that the switching off is actually a relief, I like the horse to participate in the treatment with at least a small degree of awareness. If they are falling asleep, the shiatsu will work, but you are not getting any more feedback. Also, they may begin to tip over while you are rotating a leg. One old horse client would just hear my voice in the barn and begin to relax. As soon as I began touching, he would fall asleep. This was dangerous for me, so it was his owner's job to keep him awake during his treatment. She sometimes had to tap him strongly to wake him up as he started to sink his considerable weight into my hands.

Other horses, if sore or just sensitive, may need a break from the intensity of the treatment. When working on horses with several problems, taking a break allows the energy you have helped move to circulate, without the distraction of continuing with technique after technique. Giving shiatsu allows energy to circulate for healing purposes, and sometimes the surge of this released energy, especially if it has been held tightly for a long time, may be quite stimulating. Movement allows this energy to flow and gives the horse the opportunity to move and correct his own imbalances. Otherwise, the horse may become fidgety if you continue to work.

These breaks usually entail a short walk on the lead line, either outdoors, or in an indoor arena. Sometimes I ask someone else to walk the horse so I may observe the effects of the work I have done so far. If an actual walk is not needed or if the horse is on stall rest, just leave for a few minutes, then return and proceed. Always recenter yourself after taking a break.

A break in a paddock is also appropriate at times. Watch from the fence; your horse may run around expressing the joy of released pain, leap about exuberantly, spin and rear, then stop and roll, or simply stand peacefully and meditate, or graze contentedly. Some horses are so happy and full of themselves when they suddenly realize the aches and pains are gone, they show off to prove how beautifully they move. This may be quite an interesting and beautiful display. Pay close attention to your horse's movements in terms of the meridians he is expressing or not expressing. This may give you some further treatment ideas. If you go inside the paddock with him, he is likely to follow you around asking for more touching. It will not be difficult to get him to come back for the rest of the treatment. Avoid letting him run too much as exhaustion will deplete the reserves of energy you have just tapped.

These breaks allow the horse to do his own corrective exercise. He moves in ways you cannot duplicate with shiatsu. The horse is an expert at trusting his instincts and the movements following treatment or during a break will further align and balance. Sometimes the break is necessary for the purpose of actually moving the energy more strongly than at the walk. A trot will help move the energy and show the horse that the pain may now be gone, and the movement is easy and fun. When the gait improves during a treatment break, compliment your horse on how clever he is to get better so quickly. Do not be discouraged if you do not see any immediate improvement. A chronically lame horse may not realize at first that the restriction that contributed to the lameness has been alleviated. My first experience of a case such as this was a horse who had been very lame for some months. I turned him out in the indoor arena following his first treatment. He started to walk showing the same hesitating uneven gait. As he suddenly realized the pain was gone, his face became happy and animated and he began to gallop across the arena. He stopped short in the corner and just stared at his reflection in the mirror, then ran to his owner to say thank you with many big wet kisses.

When observing your horse during a break or at the end of a treatment at liberty, try to ascertain how his movement corrects his problems. For example, rolling on each side stimulates the meridians on the sides of the body, rolling completely over also stimulates the Bladder Meridian.

Movement as Corrective Exercise

ROLLING

Rolling is an important therapeutic movement for the structure of your horse. It can help move blocked energy and rebalance ki, ease tight muscles, stimulate the nervous system (the Bladder Meridian relates to the autonomic nervous system) and realign the spine. You may have noticed a protruding or sinking-in vertebra during your work on the back. Rolling will help push the dislodged vertebra back into place. In the case of a vertebra that is sinking in, rolling gives all the other vertebrae of the spine a push and can cause the release of the vertebra that was out of alignment. Rolling is like a grand finale to your work. You have set up the situation for healing and the horse is finishing the job. You have loosened him up, stretched him out and relaxed him. He feels so good he can now express himself more comfortably. Watching horses enjoy themselves after my treatment is my reward.

One of my cases had a severe backache for months. His owner tried everything. She bought a book on massage by a well-known author but when her horse saw her coming in with the book after the first time, he hid in the corner of his stall; the techniques were too strong and painful for even this big yang Thoroughbred. In desperation, his owner lost weight and she was already very small. She really loved this horse. After the first treatment I had her walk him for me. His knees began to buckle in that characteristic prelude to the roll. She looked shocked. I assured her this was the best thing that could happen and that he was doing his corrective exercises. He rolled on each side, shook off and rolled completely over a few times. There was a huge cloud of dust around us as we watched this relieved horse. The owner had never seen her horse roll. She thought it was something he just never did. He was never dirty from rolling. After this, he began to roll frequently and, although this increased grooming time, he was happy and comfortable.

After this lovely display, we took him to his stall and watched as he fell asleep immediately. This was a perfect ending. The nap helped his energy restore itself without the distractions of the senses being awake and aware. She reported that there was no further evidence of the sore back.

TOUCHING ON THE MOVE

During breaks when someone else walks the horse, you may see an area of the horse's body where there is no energy moving, or no awareness of incorporating that area into movement to contribute to wholeness. The technique I sometimes use in these cases is simple. Walk along near the horse. Talk to him to let your presence and proximity be known, then, gently touch the area that needs the horse's notice. Keep holding as you both walk along. The first time I was inspired to use this technique was on a horse with a shoulder problem. The walk did not show the push from behind the shoulder the horse needs to balance the pull from the front. I touched the muscles just above the elbow and held gently and steadily as we walked along. The horse was able to feel this and was reminded to use these muscles. I had released their tension during treatment, now my touch increased awareness. The gait changed within about five strides. Another horse was not using his Bladder Meridian energy in his legs as he walked. I walked along holding the Bladder Meridian in one rear leg, then the other. The area I held was the fullest area of muscle between the tail and the hock. He extended his stride immediately.

REARING

After treatment, during turnout, your horse may become so enthusiastic that he displays behavior that shocks you, rearing, for example, to show a relief from pain. The full rear stretches the meridians under the belly: the Stomach Meridian, the Kidney Meridian and the Conception Vessel; perhaps you should pay these some attention during the next session.

BUCKING

Bucking stretches the back and can be either a strong expression of pain or a corrective exercise. After a treatment, it is in the category of corrective exercise if the horse is moving at will and unimpeded. Bucking stretches the Bladder Meridian and the Governing Vessel.

STRETCHING

Watch your horse stretch to determine exactly which meridians he is expressing. Observe the angle of the leg and the distance of the foot from the ground if the rear legs are being stretched. Some horses do long cat stretches. These stretch the back and back of the legs, the Bladder Meridian and Small Intestine Meridian.

These movements help your horse express wholeness rather than a collection of body parts, some of them painful. The individual corrective exercises work with the ki you have released, the ki that heals. Listen to the inner voice of the horse expressing himself.

Reactions

The nature of energy is movement and change. Every horse has a different reaction to treatment. During the session they may change from a curious and busy horse, trying to groom you in return for your attention, to a sleepy and glazed-eyed big baby. This is normal because, as you work, natural painkillers called endorphins are being released throughout the body to relax the horse. This is why a formerly hyperactive horse will become relaxed and perhaps sleepy during and after the session.

There are now many horses who have had a lot of sessions with me. These horses seem to have a relaxation response as soon as they hear my voice. They immediately respond to my first touch because their bodies are trained to receive. They are mentally conditioned to associate me with pleasurable feelings. I try not to be discouraged when a horse does not seem to be enjoying my work because of recent shoeing, worming, or too much noise in the area.

A new client asked me to work on her mare, Windy. Windy is an American Saddlebred who was abused in the course of her early training with former owners. She has many physical and emotional problems as a result of this that are taking her years to overcome. Fortunately, her present owner loves her intensely and is patient and understanding. Windy is reluctant to accept new people into her life, including me. Her back legs are forbidden and dangerous territory and, while working on her hindquarters, I must stay clear of them. Her owner must hold her during the sessions and comfort her. I had to work on her in the aisle, as she was not happy having me in her stall, even with her owner there. When she occasionally does begin to relax, she catches herself and gets nervous again. After the first session, I felt unsatisfied. Because it was such a struggle and dangerous to work on her, I wondered if I should continue to work with her myself, or teach the owner some techniques on another horse so that she should practice on Windy herself (which I also did). After the session we turned her out and she began to roll. She rolled completely over from each side, which her owner had never seen her do before. I knew then that I would continue to work directly with Windy. Windy's owner did not tell her riding instructor that Windy was having her first shiatsu session. During the lesson the instructor commented enthusiastically on how well Windy was moving and how comfortable she looked.

The third time I went to work on her, I made a mistake with the date of treatment. While I was awaiting the owner's arrival (which never came) I stood outside Windy's stable door and touched her a bit around the ears and upper neck. She alternately pinned her ears and gave me dirty looks and seemed to want me to go away. We played this game for about ten minutes before I left, thinking one of us had gotten the appointment date wrong. That night, the owner called me and said that later in the day when she arrived to visit her horse and ride, Windy was uncharacteristically relaxed and happy. She was wondering why, when one of the stable hands mentioned that I had been there waiting for her at Windy's door. It was hard for me to believe what she and Windy knew to be true: just a bit of well-placed touching can have benefits. Sometimes even I must admit that I am surprised by the extent of this beautiful work!

DELAYED REACTIONS

We do not know exactly what is happening inside the body during and after shiatsu: because of the uniqueness of each individual, reactions to treatment are varied. This is natural and normal. For example, in a horse with very slow-moving energy caused by illness, fatigue, injury, or just a natural tendency, you may not notice any change in gait after the session if you were working on this horse to improve movement. He may be relaxed and happy afterward, but there may be no noticeable change. It is entirely possible that the next day you will see a marked difference for the better. You may even see the difference show up two or three days later, so do not worry that you have not accomplished anything if the results are not immediate. Some yang types take a little longer to utilize energy, but the results will be lasting. Some yin types may react immediately in a startlingly positive way. How long they can 'hold' this change depends upon the individual.

Treating Kyo and Jitsu

The words 'kyo' and 'jitsu' describe the distortion, or imbalance, of energy, or ki, within the meridian lines. When speaking of imbalance, we are referring to 'misplaced energy', energy that needs to redistribute itself to regain balance. Balance is the ability to cope with a wide range of challenging situations.

Kyo is hypo, jitsu is hyper. Indentations along meridian lines are kyo, protrusions are jitsu. Some points need to be more yin or yang, according to their functions, but if a point or area is excessively yin, it becomes kyo, if it is excessively yang, it becomes jitsu. The kyo areas need to be patiently nurtured and tonified, the jitsu areas can take stronger techniques because they need to be sedated. Some points in relation to their location in the body may feel kyo or jitsu. For example, the area just past the withers, toward the tail, may sink in a bit on some horses anatomically and areas just past large muscle groups may also sink in naturally. Do not confuse these places with kyo areas (although they may, in fact, actually be kyo). Use the energetic manifestations as your guide for determining kyo and jitsu. Some large muscle groups may feel jitsu by their structural nature. Consider the energetic response to determine if they are jitsu.

MUSCULAR BALANCE AND THE RESULTS OF MUSCULAR IMBALANCE

Consider the actual muscle type of the horse (*see* The Yin Horse page 230 and The Yang Horse page 231). A healthy, well-balanced muscle that is at rest should feel pliable and firm but not tight, hard, hot and rigid. There should be no knots or lumps, stringy rubber-band-like areas or tension. The bundles of muscle tissue you see in a horse during work should not be evident at rest. If there is a specific and chronic area of muscle tension that is not able to be released when at rest, consider the meridian that goes through the area. If the tension does not eventually release, the energy in the meridian may be affected.

For example, if the horse has a chronic pain in one area of the back that goes into spasm and stays that way for long periods of time, the meridian associated with the point, as well as the energy in the entire Bladder Meridian, can be affected. The point that relates to the Lung Meridian that is on the Bladder Meridian (Bl 13) is just behind the withers on both sides, and if there is an injury in the area of the Lung Meridian that does not heal for any reason, the Lung Meridian and perhaps the actual lungs may suffer. Or, if a chronic muscle spasm actually pulls the vertebrae out of alignment, if nature and shiatsu, or another modality, do not encourage the realignment of the vertebrae, the energy flow of the entire body will be affected. This is another reason why it is so important to consider and treat the entire body, rather than just the symptoms. Working on meridian lines allows the body to adjust itself. If energy is in balance, the bone structure can move into proper alignment.

It is easier to find the jitsu areas because they are obvious to the touch and sometimes visually apparent. They feel warm, hot, tight, hard, active or busy, with energy either stuck or vibrating within and not moving in either direction. Techniques that sedate the jitsu are strong quick pressure, large rotations and big stretches held to maximum tension and, also, working quickly and with firm pressure along meridian lines. Jitsu areas are relatively easy to sedate in a healthy individual whose life force is fairly unimpeded by stress, both physically and mentally.

The kyo is harder to find because it is subtle, hidden, and perhaps very deep within. Kyo is more difficult to treat because it represents such a depleted condition, often exacerbated by the fatigue of chronic conditions. Upon palpation, it feels cool or cold, tired, unresponsive and lacking in energy. Your hand may feel pulled into the body. These very kyo points must be held patiently to get warmth and nurturing energy to go deeply into the body. Techniques that address kyo are gentle holding and working slowly along the meridian lines.

A yin type horse is usually prone to kyo conditions, a yang type horse is usually prone to more jitsu conditions. Avoid sedating the kyo horse as whatever remaining energy he has will be consumed, causing the condition to worsen. It is particularly important to tonify the kyo in this depleted horse, and the jitsu will take care of itself. This theory was developed by Master Shizuto Masunaga. In this way we treat the cause without attacking the symptom. Working only on the jitsu, as done by some Asian bodywork techniques, may get results but they may be only temporary. Kyo is the cause, jitsu is the symptom. If we are successful in finding and treating the cause, which is depleted energy, the symptoms disappear. The earlier we are able to do this, the better chance we have of success. The longer the condition is allowed to persist, the closer it gets to western medicine being able to name it. Shiatsu treats the whole individual to support innate good health. It is best for maintaining vitality and good health, therefore preventing dis-ease, and disease.

Just as there are yin and yang type horses, there are yin or yang type conditions. In this style of shiatsu we are looking for the kyo, which is the underlying cause of the jitsu. Again, this is the theory of the late Master Shizuto Masunaga. Kyo points or areas feel as if there is little or no energy moving through. The point itself may cause your hand to feel that it is drawn inward as this emptiness that is kyo wants to receive energy. It is said that nature hates a vacuum. There is something lacking, a need, an unfulfilled desire to be more alive, that is kyo. It may take several minutes of working the meridian which the point is on, while concentrating particularly on holding the kyo point, to finally feel some energy response. Treating the kyo takes patience and perseverance and a letting go of the ego. In working with the kyo horse, you must be patient. The underlying kyo can take a long time to come back to a normal condition. Do not give too long a treatment as excessive stimulation could further deplete your horse's energy. More than forty-five minutes may be too much. Gradually acclimatize your kyo depleted horse to treatment. You will be methodically helping to build up the energy reserves needed to maintain radiant good health. Yin horses experiencing chronic kyo conditions are susceptible to reinjury and relapse into illness, so make rest and top quality food priorities. You may find some herbs will help as well.

Treating the jitsu condition with sedation is easier but, unless you work with the kyo places, the symptoms will return. Sedation techniques include strong pressure and big movements. The fingertips and elbows are more sedating than the palms. You can work more quickly and with more pressure which can be very specific. You must work with confidence. If you can accomplish this while relaxing your horse, jitsu energy has a better chance of dispersing itself into kyo points, or perhaps just dispersing. Jiggling is a dispersion technique, so are stretching and percussion. Big sustained stretches will help disperse the overaccumulation of energy that is jitsu. Stretch to the first point of resistance, hold a few seconds, release an inch or two, and stretch a bit further before releasing.

Yin horses may have jitsu conditions and yang horses may have kyo conditions. It is important when treating a yin horse with a jitsu condition to work carefully so as not to sedate too much and thus deplete energy. Sedate only the jitsu areas you find, not the whole horse. Treating kyo conditions in yang horses is easier, as they have a good supply of energy that gives them a great potential to overcome imbalances. **Balanced energy is both the cause and effect of radiant good health.**

A good example of kyo and jitsu conditions within one problem is the common cold. A cold with running eyes, clear and abundant mucus coming from the nostrils, of very long duration with ensuing fatigue and susceptibility to relapse (Chinese medicine states 'beware of the cold, because it leads to all diseases') is a yin cold. A cold with congested eyes, blocked tear ducts, thick mucus that can also smell, fever and lung congestion, is a yang cold. The symptoms may be severe but the duration is short.

Your technique will become more effective as you become better able to determine kyo and jitsu.

AN EXAMPLE OF HOW TO TREAT KYO AND JITSU ON THE BACK

You are working along the Bladder Meridian on the back with your supporting hand across the withers. A few inches past the withers you find a jitsu area. Your horse gives you a 'look' and you feel heat coming from the area. You do not dwell on the area, only make note of it. Further along, perhaps near the hindquarters, you feel a kyo spot that sinks in, and has no energetic response. Move your supporting hand to the jitsu and hold the kyo with your other hand. In a few seconds, you will probably feel these areas change. Typically, the jitsu releases and becomes more pliable, and the kyo area fills up with energy, which you begin to feel moving or pulsing. Hold these points a few seconds more, then proceed with your chosen technique. As you work along the back, stay longer in the kyo places, where your palm or fingertips sink in. Hold there until you feel a filling up or pulse of energy under your hand. This may take a few seconds, or up to half a minute. What you have just experienced is a redistribution of energy, the innate ability of the body, with a bit of help, to balance itself. If you have actually found the most kyo and most jitsu you will be able to accomplish this. You may find a secondary kyo and jitsu on the back. These will respond as well. Sometimes by treating the primary kyo and jitsu, the secondary ones will take care of themselves. You are communicating with the body in a very basic but sophisticated way, you are touching life.

Because of the overuse of a horse, any injury that is not completely healed along a meridian line can be the eventual cause of an organ problem. Conversely, a chronic organ problem can cause the meridian to be out of balance and lead to structural misalignment.

While working with kyo and jitsu, it is important to remember that we are manipulating the energy of another being. Do so respectfully, and with a reverent attitude. We are touching life!

Manifestations of Sensation in the Points, from Normal to Painful

There are varying degrees of point sensitivity along the meridians throughout your horse's body; the range is wide. Here are some possible manifestations: numb, ticklish, comfortable, pleasurable, pleasurably painful, comfortably painful, downright painful. An experienced practitioner may know by touch alone what the horse is feeling within a wide range of sensations. Learn what normal and healthy feel like before attempting to determine imbalance, kyo and jitsu. It is crucial to know if a point is going to be painful before you cause the horse a pain that will make him lose confidence in you and move away from the pain.

NORMAL

A point where energy is moving as it should feels comfortable for the horse; it will have a very noticeable quality to your touch. It could be described as uninteresting because it does not attract your attention in any way, it feels normal. The point feels pliable and alive. When you greet it with your touch and a medium amount of pressure, it greets you back. It does not suck you in and it does not push you away. It has healthy elasticity. If you hold it for a few seconds, you will feel a smoothness to its energy immediately. There may be no visible change in the horse because everything is where it should be, or you may get a relaxation response.

ABNORMAL

If the point is numb and lacking in all sensitivity, you may feel it as dead, unresponsive, thick like dense foam rubber. It has no energetic response as you hold it. You could hold it for an hour and get no response because you must first work on the meridian throughout the body on both sides, and then check again for feeling. It may be the location of an old injury, or chronic irritation from the saddle. If you suspect an old injury, be patient in getting energy to move through this area; it may take months of treatments.

If the point is ticklish your horse may get a bit jumpy, but not as he would from pain. The jumpiness is a bit hyper, almost giddy, and the horse may begin nibbling you and playing with anything at hand. This ticklishness is a manifestation of jitsu, too much energy in the area. Look for a corresponding kyo and hold the two points with steady palm pressure until you feel energy moving between your hands.

The nature of energy is change and movement.

Practitioners and Other Treatments

If you feel another, perhaps more experienced, practitioner or therapist, or a different type of treatment, is advisable for a patient, then do your homework first.

HOW TO CHOOSE A PRACTITIONER

Any practitioner you choose should be comfortable answering the following questions:

- Where, and for how long, did you study?
- With whom did you study, and what are the qualifications of your teacher?
- How long have you been in practice?
- Would you give me referrals?
- What types of problems do you specialize in?
- How many sessions will it take for me to see a positive change?
- Do you have experience with my horse's particular problem?

Do not be afraid to ask questions. You do not even have to make an appointment the first time you speak to a potential therapist.

Any practitioner should allow you to observe them work and answer your questions afterward. They should be comfortable around horses and use safe handling practices. If the person is not competent they can hurt your horse or be seriously hurt.

There are short courses available that will get a practitioner started. I have heard of weekend courses in massage that certify people who are not equipped to handle any real problems. These people should spend a lot of time practicing on their own and friends' horses before going out in the real world of horses with problems.

My own Level 1 course teaches (in three days) a good thorough full-body session for the horse, but I ask my students to explain to the people whose horses they are required to practice on that they are beginners, not experts.

OTHER TREATMENTS

Ask your vet for referrals. Many vets these days are doing acupuncture and are open to other modalities.

Lameness, back pain, weak hindquarters and other physical problems as well as many behavior problems can be helped, and possibly cured, by well-trained practitioners of bodywork therapies but these same problems could be made worse by inadequately trained people. Chiropractic, massage therapy, shiatsu, etc., there is a wide range of possible modalities to choose from. Although, for obvious reasons, shiatsu is my favorite modality, there are times when I choose another type of practitioner for myself and my horse, dog and people clients.

Massage

Racehorses seem to do very well when treated with massage therapy because their stress is primarily muscular and they are stressing the same muscles over and over again, usually without any other activity and limited turnout time. Of course, they have emotional stresses as well. I have never found anyone who worked with racehorses who was willing to take the time to learn a few shiatsu techniques to help the horses after I left. Shiatsu gives horses too much to think about, and they may become too deeply relaxed to care about winning. A good general all-over sports massage will be best.

Chiropractic

Shiatsu will help misaligned bones adjust themselves in time, but sometimes the pain is too stressful to wait. It would be appropriate to call in a chiropractor and get things moving while doing shiatsu as well. The shiatsu treatment should not be given the same day as chiropractic.

Work with a chiropractor who is also a vet, or a human care practitioner who has been certified by the American Veterinary Chiropractic Association in Hillsdale, Illinois. In other countries, try to locate an equivalent organization. Chiropractors should only use their hands or a hand-held 'activator' which administers a quick light tap and is painless. The use of ropes, mallets, and other contraptions is dangerous.

Acupuncture

Acupuncture is helpful for horses who have been so severely traumatized that they are unable to allow themselves to be touched. It will also help for equine diseases and nervous-system disorders. It is a wonderful adjunct to shiatsu.

Note If a practitioner is performing a technique that is stressing your horse physically and mentally, you have the right and responsibility to express your concern and ask them to stop immediately. I have seen horses with problems that resulted from their owners being too afraid or shy to speak out when they saw something happening during some treatments other than shiatsu. Trust your instincts. Protect your horse.

Gaining Experience

If you wish to pursue shiatsu with horses beyond the treatment of just your own horse, here is some advice: become very comfortable with these techniques on your own horse, and try to practice daily. Perfect the basic techniques, e.g. working the Bladder Meridian on the back, leg rotations and stretches, and some neck work. If possible, take my courses as well as any courses in bodywork for horses that are available in your area. I do not recommend combining modalities but sometimes a technique from a different modality is appropriate during a shiatsu session. It is also important to know what is available in order to help others find a suitable course of action with which to help horses with problems.

After you have spent some time gaining experience, flow, confidence and effectiveness, ask your friends if you might practice on their horses. These practice horses should be relatively free of serious problems, although some stiffness in the muscles and joints will teach you a lot, and you will help these horses. Do not overtreat a horse the first time, and always let a few days elapse before giving the second treatment. It is likely that a sore horse could be a bit more sensitive the day after the treatment and you should make the owner aware of that eventuality.

If you have taken some courses already, you could go to horse facilities and offer your services. Tell them you are a beginner and not a professional. Working on school horses is a tremendous learning experience, and they will really appreciate your attention. Go to horse shows and study the horses and riders; look for meridian distortions, imbalances in movement and the body language of the riders. If you think a horse desperately needs your attention, be careful, as most horse owners will resent a stranger telling them their horse is sore, unhappy, out of balance or lame. Also, if eventually you work professionally with horses as a shiatsu practitioner, be discreet, do not tell your horse clients' owners who your other horse clients are, unless you have permission.

All my horse clients have come to me via word of mouth. There is nothing so valuable as the recommendation of an owner whose horse you have helped. When you have worked with a horse a few times, give the owner a gift certificate to pass on to someone who may need it. This will help others learn about you. With shiatsu as your work, and love in your hands, you are bound to do a lot of good.

Case Studies

Student practitioner   Tracy Bleaken – Level One

Horse Frosty – twenty-year-old Welsh Cross gelding, 13.2 hh
Work hacking, fun rides
Owner Gill West (signed and completed Permission and Evaluation form)

History

Gill has owned Frosty for twelve years and has known him all his life. Frosty has mainly been used for hacking and fun rides. He lives on a hillside and has recently been finding it hard to walk down the hills, shuffling his hind legs and dragging his toes.

Personality

Frosty is a yang horse, being stocky, outgoing and active.

Session One 3/2/–

Visual observation

Watching and mimicking Frosty, I felt his back was not swinging, and when he stood still he was tucking his hind legs under his body to arch his back.

Observation by touch

While stroking, I felt Frosty's back was warm and tender, I also noticed he had a raised vertebra under the saddle area which Gill told me had been evident for some time, and a chiropractor had told her it would always be present. I began by working very lightly along the Bladder Meridian to warm the back. Gill told me that Frosty suffered from sweet itch in the summer and was sensitive about his back and tail being touched, I explained that this work may also help to desensitise him. I jiggled the neck, the muscles were tense; I jiggled the forelegs and these muscles were also tense. I began light stretches forwards and began rotations but kept them small as I felt some resistance. I rested Frosty's hind hooves on his toes and jiggled but, again, the muscles were tight. At this point Frosty became a little restless, so I decided to take a break. While Frosty stood and ate his hay, I explained to Gill that he may need to rest and readjust himself a little.

About ten minutes later I began again by stroking Frosty who seemed more relaxed. I worked lightly along the Bladder Meridian again and his back felt less arched. I began percussion on his hindquarter muscles and showed Gill this technique and also how to work along Bladder Meridian.

Session Two – 9/2/–

Frosty looked more relaxed as I began stroking, standing quietly in his stable. I worked the Bladder Meridian and felt Frosty's back to be cooler and lower. I jiggled his forelegs and the rotations were easier. I began work behind and in front of his shoulders which were quite tight in front so I did not work too deeply. When I jiggled the hind legs the muscles looked softer and Gill told me she had been using percussion when she groomed. When I stroked his tail, Frosty clamped it to his bottom but, as I carried on stroking, Frosty began to relax so I used light stretches from side to side, stroked and finished. I showed Gill how to stroke and stretch Frosty's tail sideways to accustom him to it being handled. After this session Frosty was turned out and went for a trot around.

Session Three – 16/2/–

I began with stroking and the rotations had become easier. I jiggled his neck and the muscles were flexible. I began lateral neck flexes and did these around my body as I felt that, with Frosty being small, I would be at a wrong angle if using palm pressure; his neck was flexible. I jiggled his hind legs, the muscles were softer, and began tail work. Frosty accepted my touch so I rotated each individual vertebra and then used a full stretch to finish which Frosty leant into and groaned. I used percussion on the large muscles, stroked and finished. While stroking at the end, I noticed that the raised vertebra had settled. I explained to Gill that I thought this raised vertebra had caused Frosty to have difficulty walking and was the reason he was arching his back.

Conclusion

Frosty is now back to his old self, whizzing about and being very naughty in, according to Gill, his normal way. Whenever I visit Frosty he seems happy to see me and Gill asked if I would clip him for her. I did this one day while she was at work; she arrived at the yard late and was surprised to find him finished and back in his field. Gill explained that, before, he always had to be sedated to be clipped.

I have learned from working with Frosty that shiatsu is a good way to communicate with horses and, because of the communication, they readily accept other things, however alien, we ask of them.

Owner's comments

Frosty is now back to his usual self, full of energy and enthusiasm, after a time of feeling stiff and uncomfortable.

Student practitioner   John Brooks

Horse Orson – nineteen-year-old crossbred gelding, 15.1 hh
Work Slow hacking
Owner Jo Morgan

History

Jo Morgan has owned Orson for four years. Vets say he has chronic obstructive pulmonary disease (COPD), a cough condition like asthma. He is given herbal medicine, though vets are talking of using a nebuliser. His condition is always the same, winter or summer. When out, the first trot leads to a coughing fit then he clears his nostrils and after that is OK. The discharge is a fine moisture/vapour. He has a very greasy/dirty coat and a skin rash, usually on the left side of shoulder. He eats well but is not very active. If other horses run round the field, Orson watches. He tends to be on his own; he likes company but not close and does not groom the other horses.

Personality
Orson is very willing to please and well mannered.

Session One – 13/4/99

Visual observation

Head held low in walk, tight lower neck, full torso, loose forelegs and buttocks. Discharge from eyes. Very clear ridge on Large Intestine line in neck.

Observation by touch

All the above confirmed. Stiff in upper shoulder/lower neck. Twitchy withers.

There was an immediate and strong connection on the Bladder line and gurgling innards. Mainly kyo under the saddle area, loose in buttocks. I worked neck Bladder, Gall Bladder and Small Intestine. Orson was restless and mildly annoyed when I worked on Large Intestine, stamping his foot at one point. All indicators point to Large Intestine (Metal): asthma, skin issues, poor coat, nasal discharge, boundaries with others, introvert.

There were good turns for leg stretches but it was hard when turning the lower neck: I used dispersing techniques. I also followed the Large Intestine line and Lung line in chest/lower leg. Great forward stretches with loud relieving clicks.

Orson appreciated the face sequence: orbital ridges and tear ducts.

Both Orson and I lost concentration when the yard became busy and he wanted his food. I stopped after the usual routine. Jo Morgan, who watched the whole session, was most appreciative.

Three days later I saw Jo who said that Orson had actually trotted to her when called from the field, moving with the others. 'This', she said 'is a first, so something's happening'.

Session Two – 20/4/99

Orson appears in the yard lively and trotting immediately behind the three other horses being brought in. He is a spritely old fellow and looks good. There is no discharge from the nostrils and less from the eyes. He still has a careworn look about him – Eeyore type – but he is content and steady. I am less drawn to the Large Intestine groove which is less pronounced. However the Bladder lines under the saddle area look extremely kyo and so they prove.

I concentrated on this section with a focused intensity. I worked both lines with the palm heel then the fingers and thumb, and even the elbow. One area felt like a deep well that I could sink into up to my armpit. Orson was motionless except for the odd shudder which ran up his neck, or a deep sigh which seemed to move the other way to the tail. I also tried to pick out key Bladder points like Bl 23 and the Large Intestine yu points. I felt a strong and vibrant activity.

I followed the Bladder line down and also worked the yin side exploring both Kidney and Liver. He tolerated a full sequence of rotations and stretches on the hind legs and was flexible.

The Stomach line on the hip seemed kyo but he kept moving away from the touch so I started neck and face work. I worked Large Intestine which was jitsu so I followed the line quickly and actively to the hooves. I also tried Gall Bladder in his neck and shoulder which sent a distinct shiver/twitch through to the hip.

Orson loves the face routine: the nasal passages, nostrils, mouth, prominent jaw bones, Stomach line, Large Intestine line, orbital ridges, Gall Bladder and Triple Heater points. Followed Triple Heater round the ears and down the neck on both sides. That connection was good and I recalled a characteristic of Triple Heater being a tendency to being uncomfortable with groups/in company; perhaps, although I still feel the concentration on Metal and Water is right.

Orson is such a patient horse. The eye contact is long and comfortable. He accepts the head sequence without any resistance. He is a pleasure to work with.

Session Three – 5/5/99

Again I was drawn to the Bladder line and Stomach line outer hip area both of which appeared kyo and proved to be when touched. Also, the Large Intestine line in the neck was prominent. There was no discharge from the nostrils and minimal discharge from the eyes.

I worked the Bladder line slowly and found deep kyo areas in the saddle area. He settled into the touch with ease. I worked both the upper and secondary line on the torso then moved down the rear leg. Here I explored the yin side and the points around the hoof. I was drawn to Liver, and particularly Liver 3.

He was less comfortable with the work on the kyo areas around the hip stamping his foot down hard on the opposite side at one point, which for Orson is like a tantrum, but he settled as I soothed him with touch and voice and he allowed me to continue.

On the chest and forelegs the focus was on Lung and Large Intestine but I also acknowledged the Fire meridians to help add a bit of spark into the proceedings. Heart Protector (Constrictor) saw the strongest connection which indicated a balancing in one-to-one relationships.

The Metal element meridians of Lung and Large Intestine are key to the breathing/asthma imbalances and it was the Lung points in the chest which provided the kyo areas. Even though they are not always easily accessible on Orson, the points were clear and well received.

I acknowledged the Large Intestine in the neck and face but I was not drawn to stay long. In fact I got the impression that at the end of a hot spring day it was time to end calmly.

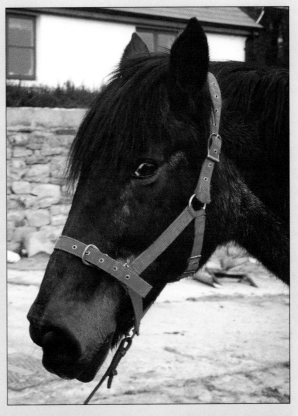

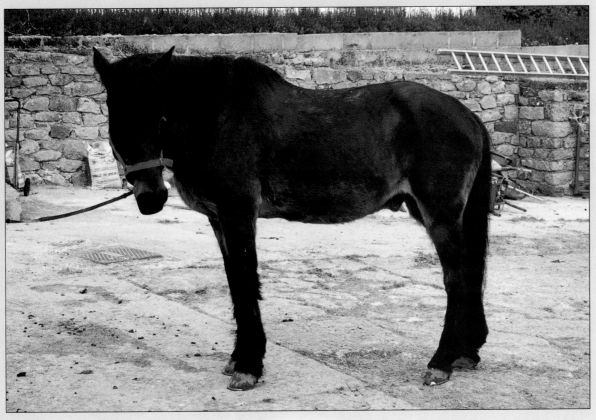

Student practitioner   Vivienne Isaac – Level Three

Horse Ginga – three-year-old Thoroughbred chestnut filly, 15.1 hh
Work None as yet, unbroken
Owner Julie Hibbitt

History

Whilst in her box, Ginga became cast and sustained severe trauma to the nearside radial nerve, consequently displaying classic symptoms of radial nerve damage. On veterinary advice she was placed on twelve weeks box rest, the owner being advised that the prognosis in such cases is usually poor. The owner also sought advice from a qualified physiotherapist who suggested electrotherapy twice daily.

Ginga's condition continued to deteriorate with the muscles over the scapula wasting away, and the toe of the affected leg being seriously worn down as it was dragged with every movement.

At this point the prognosis was extremely poor, and the next option was to either have the filly destroyed, or try to regain the use of the shoulder. This is when Julie got in touch with me and asked me to see if there was anything I could do.

Personality
Temperamental and aggressive.

Session One – 16/7/98
Visual observation
Her entire body was tense with holding herself on three legs and dragging the other one along. There was no muscle at all over the left shoulder with the shoulder blade visible through the skin. Her overall condition was poor as she had little appetite. She has been handled very little and Julie warned me to beware of her kicking and biting.

Observation by touch
Under the circumstances it is understandable that the filly's attitude was somewhat temperamental and aggressive initially, but she accepted my touch.

After the introduction and all-over stroking, I used the following techniques: palmed the Bladder Meridian from the withers to the croup, followed by finger pressure; palmed over the withers and in front and behind the shoulders, starting on the good side; palm and finger pressure along the Small Intestine, Triple Heater and Large Intestine channels; moving-muscle technique over the quarters to help release the tension here; palm and finger pressure along the Bladder and Gall Bladder in the quarters and hind leg; very gentle rotation of the nearside foreleg and hoof (as she was not able to stand on this leg, no other leg rotations or stretches were possible or appropriate); concluded with all-over stroking.

I worked the Small Intestine, Triple Heater and Large Intestine as they run through the affected area, Bladder to settle her to my touch and for her all-over wellbeing, and the Gall Bladder to help reduce muscle soreness.

Ginga settled well to the session, I had to beware of her nipping but she never offered to kick. By the end of the session she was holding a lot less tension throughout her whole body and was able to move a little more easily.

Session Two – 21/7/98
There was a clear improvement in Ginga's general look and she was a lot less tense all over. I followed a very similar session procedure to that of the first session, adding in palming the three lines of the neck as the Large Intestine, Small Intestine and Triple Heater channels also run along the neck.

When we walked her out at the end of this session she was able to use her near foreleg more easily, and it was less inclined to bend over and drag.

Session Three – 27/7/98
Again, Ginga had maintained the improvement since the previous session and she was bearing

more weight on the nearside fore.

As well as working the Bladder, Small Intestine, Triple Heater and Gall Bladder Meridians, I was able to jiggle her hind legs. Although she was clearly feeling better she was still quick to nip me if I was not careful when I was within reach, so I wet my hand and swished round her top and bottom gums – she was not quite sure what to make of that.

At the end of this third session she was able to walk much more normally.

I continued with a further three sessions. By the end of the fourth she was sound in walk, and almost sound in trot by the end of the sixth. The later sessions were a little shorter and I used more rotations and stretches, as she was able to bear weight on all four legs. I suggested to Julie that she needed to be walked out several times a day to build up the muscles over her shoulders. The vet also suggested this.

I showed Julie the all-over stroking and palming techniques to use on her forelegs. She did admit to me that unfortunately she never had time to do them. (She co-runs the family business with her husband, has three children, about six horses and various other animals to look after so it was hardly surprising!)

Conclusion

The most important thing I learned from working with this horse was not to underestimate the benefits of shiatsu. I have to say that I was sceptical about being able to help this horse when I first saw her. The difference amazed me. I have to admit that I did not write up this case study straight away, as I just did not expect such a spectacular improvement. Another point was that conditions were far from ideal, with a noisy six-year-old constantly interrupting, the telephone ringing and dogs barking. I did get the little boy to work on his Shetland pony, but the only thing he really wanted to do was pull its tail!

Nine months after the treatment (when the photo was taken) Ginga had just started work. It is a shame I do not have 'before and after' photographs. Fifteen months on from her treatment she is enjoying being ridden out regularly and is quiet and easy to handle.

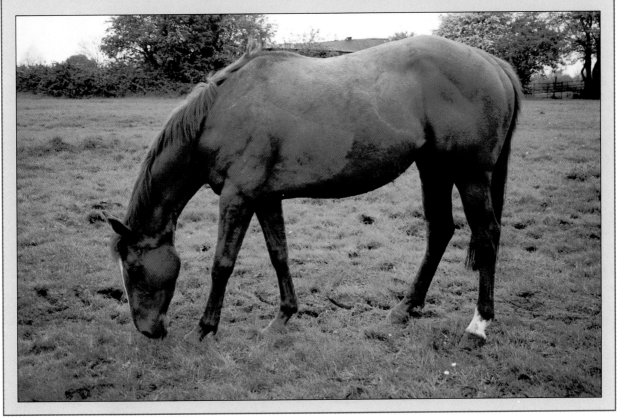

Student practitioner   Roberta Cormack-Brown – Level Three

Horse Dylan – eight-year-old Irish-bred chestnut gelding, 14.2 hh
Work Light hacking
Owner Margaret Currie (signed and completed Permission and Evaluation form)

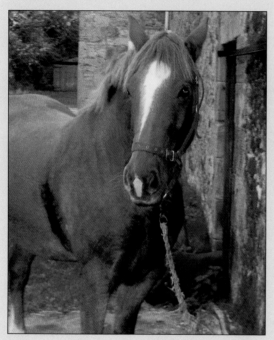

History

Margaret has had Dylan since he was two. He was bought for her two daughters to ride purely for pleasure. At the age of five he took part in the common riding (an old tradition in Scottish border towns). After one of these rides, his back legs were swollen and hot up to the hock. He was rested for six months and was given bute in his feed. When he was ridden for the first after this period of rest, he soon became lame again and, unfortunately, he has been lame off and on ever since. Arthritis has now set in.

Personality

Dylan has a nice quiet temperament. He does not object to anything you do with him, he is totally trusting. He has no vices and will do whatever is asked of him, even if he is in pain. He loves his food and tends to be a bit greedy.

Session One – 2/10/-

Visual observation

At the walk Dylan is very stiff in the hind legs, he throws his right hind leg out at the hock, away from his body, in a kind of circular movement. He has a bone spavin at the side of his right hock due to arthritis and a hollow in this thigh due to no muscle tone. He has the typical nodding action of the head which becomes more pronounced when asked to move faster. Apart from his right thigh, he looks a yang type, very strong and sturdy.

Observation through touch

Dylan felt relaxed and I did not feel tension. His legs did not feel as tight or as tense as I had expected. There was some heat in his right fetlock. He did not object to me touching his back legs or the spavin.

Dylan stood quietly during the session and relaxed into the session. He did not fuss and was not restless. Halfway through the session he looked like he was enjoying it. He did not object to his hind legs being lifted and rotated.

My techniques and procedure were: stroking, rotations, stretches, palm and finger pressure, and Bladder and Gall Bladder Meridians. I stroked all over his body and legs, then moved to Bladder Meridian and did light heel-of-palm pressure all along this meridian to the hind foot. I then did moving muscle on the hindquarters. I did the shoulders and neck, then hind leg rotations and stretches but not a full stretch. I then did tail stroking and rotations and sideways stretches, finishing with a full spinal stretch and long strokes on both sides of his body and legs.

I worked on these specific points: termination point of Bladder Meridian; Gall Bladder 21 and 44.

At the end of the session Dylan looked relaxed and happier. His owner walked him round for me and his movement looked freer, the nodding of his head was not so pronounced and he was not as reluctant to walk out. He was still throwing his right hind leg out and away from him.

Sessions Two and Three – 9/10/– and 16/10/–

In the second session I did Gall Bladder 21 an 44. His leg stretches were easier and by the third session I was able to do a full stretch of his hind legs. The rotations were also easier. There was still slight heat in his fetlock.

Conclusion

I did not develop any new techniques with Dylan, because of his arthritis I did not want to do anything that would aggravate the condition. I did the techniques and meridians which we covered in Level 2 and *Touching Horses.*

Margaret felt that the rotations and stretches helped prepare Dylan for riding and loosened him up, which made him look and feel less stiff when walking out. She also felt Dylan was benefiting from this and getting stronger in the hindlegs. I taught Margaret stroking, shoulder and hind leg rotations and stretches.

Owner's comments

My horse has arthritis in the offside hind hock and this has caused muscle wastage and made him very lame with a distorted action. After Roberta worked on him for a few sessions his lameness wore off quicker and his action behind became less distorted and more fluent. He seems happier.

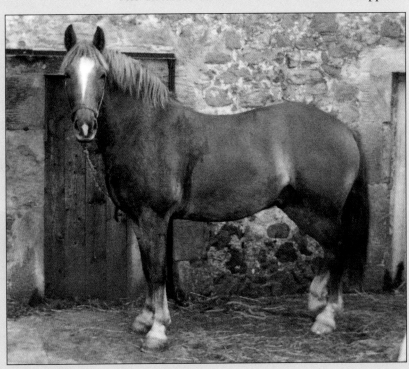

Student practitioner   Alison Croft – Level Three

Horse Swift-wind – eight-year-old Connemara cross, dapple grey gelding
Work Showjumping and general hacking
Owner Linda and Katie Roe (signed and completed Permission and Evaluation form)

History

Swift was bought from a riding school, he belonged to the owner's son who used him for affiliated showjumping. Katie has owned Swift for a year and competes in showjumping and cross-country with him.

Personality

Swift is a very nervous pony but is nice natured as well. He is responsive to people who are gentle and kind to him.

Session One – 12/8/98
Visual observation (using skills from Level 2)
When walking, Swift looks very stiff and does not use himself properly. He is stiff in both his hindquarters and his shoulders. Swift's shoulders are very heavily muscled and he seems to pull his whole weight along by them. Swift has a very long

back and appears to have a lump of muscle just behind the saddle area on both sides – this is more developed to the left than to the right. His hindquarters are solid and he wiggles in the middle at the walk. Swift does not track up and it is like watching two different horses move, one from the front and the other from the back.

Observation through touch

Swift did not want to be touched at all, at first he was very tense and shrank away from me. I stroked him gently to try and relax him and eventually he let me move in closer. I could feel tenseness throughout his body and this was more noticeable to the right. His neck, shoulder region and the area behind the saddle through his hindquarters were warm and also solid, while the saddle area was cold and hollow, this was more noticeable to the right. The top of the right-hand back leg was also cold and Swift was not happy about his lower legs being touched, both fore and hind, and kept fidgeting when I tried to touch them. Swift was not happy about his face being touched at all and was quite tense in his tail.

I used the following meridians.

Bladder I used this meridian for the physical associations of nervousness, hind-leg soreness and stiffness, headaches, neck pain, back pain and a clamped tail. The emotional associations that I noticed were fear of going into a new environment, reluctance to move forward and a tendency to be headstrong. This meridian also affects all the other meridians.

Kidney The physical association for this meridian was lumber pain, mainly due to the fact that Swift has such a long back. The emotional association was fear.

Small Intestine I used this meridian for its emotional associations. Swift has a tendency to overexert himself and overdo things, he is also overreactive and unhappy about relationships, horse or human.

Heart Same emotional associations as the Small Intestine.

Gall Bladder I used this meridian for the physical associations of general muscle soreness especially in the hind limbs, headaches and neck tension. The emotional associations were mental inflexibility, stubbornness and anger.

Liver The physical association for this meridian was hind-leg stiffness. The emotional associations were the same as the Gall Bladder.

Swift responded very well to this meridian work and by the third session his flexibility and range of movement had increased.

I applied the following specific techniques and session procedure but did not use any specific points.

Greeting I talked to Swift keeping my body low until I could get him to relax.

Stroking I stroked Swift all over slowly and gently, allowing him to relax with each point before moving on to the next.

Bladder Meridian I used palm then finger pressure from the wither area to the top of the back legs, following on down the back legs.

Kidney Meridian I used finger pressure down the inside of his hind legs.

Small Intestine Meridian I used finger pressure along the full length of this meridian and pressed around his hooves and heels.

Heart Meridian I used finger pressure on the inside of his forelegs and pressed around his hooves.

Gall Bladder Meridian I used palm pressure along the full length of this meridian.

Liver Meridian I used finger pressure along the inside of his hind legs.

Hindquarters I used holding, elbow pressure, squeezed down the hamstrings and percussed the heavily muscled areas. I then jiggled at the hock to check for looseness.

Hoof rotations With toe on floor (introduced in second and third sessions).

Neck I used neck rocking and percussion to loosen the muscles in the neck and to move energy.

Shoulders I used the blade of my hand to loosen both the front and the back of the shoulder blade. I then jiggled at the knee to check for looseness.

Tail First I stroked the tail, then did a small rotation to the left and right, a push up and pull down, walked the tail to the left and right, full tail rotation to both the left and right and a couple of full tail stretches.

Face I worked very gently with Swift's face but eventually managed to press round his eyes, down his tear ducts, go gently into his nostrils and press around them and go into his mouth and pull his cheeks down and press round his gums. *Close* I stroked Swift all over and grounded him on each leg to finish the session. I thanked Swift for the session and left him to relax in his stable.

Swift was very nervous to begin with and it took me quite a while just to get close to him. The stroking began to relax him and he enjoyed his Bladder Meridian being touched although he was very tense around his hindquarters. He began to yawn and close his eyes. Swift was not happy at first about his lower legs being touched and kept lifting them up but relaxed after a while when he realized that this was not what I wanted. Work on the Small Intestine and Heart Meridians really relaxed Swift and he leant into me for more pressure. The Gall Bladder and Liver Meridian work only seemed to relax Swift further: he lent into my pressure and stood very still, yawning and sighing. The body work went very well: Swift's tight muscles relaxed and he became a lot easier to work on. After work on the hindquarters Swift did a big arching stretch and a yawn. He was tense with the tail work to begin with but relaxed after the first rotations; Swift really enjoyed the full stretches once he realized what I wanted. Swift is very head-shy so the face work was a bit difficult but once Swift realized I was not going to hurt him he let me work on his face and relaxed. Swift seemed to enjoy the shiatsu session and found it relaxing once he realized I was not going to hurt him.

We left Swift in his stable for about ten minutes, then Katie walked him out for me. He was more relaxed than at the beginning of the session and his stride was longer and less hurried. Katie left Swift in his stable to ride later. When I next came round to see Swift about ten minutes later he was lying down resting. Katie said that when she rode him later in the day he was very laid back.

Session Two (19/8/98) and Session Three (27/8/98)

During the three sessions, Swift gradually became more relaxed and receptive to the shiatsu sessions. He was more relaxed through his body, and was more supple through his neck, shoulders and hindquarters. Swift's lower legs became easier to touch and he allowed me to press all around the top of his hooves without picking his feet up. I was also able to introduce some hoof rotations with his toe on the floor in the second and third sessions. Swift also got used to me touching his head and ears and as long as I was gentle with him he did not shy away.

I showed Katie how to stroke Swift all over to get him used to being touched. I then showed her how to work on Swift's face so that he would not be so head-shy and how to work on his tail including rotations and stretches to help the relaxation of his back. I also showed her how to press around Swift's hooves so that he would not think he would always have to pick them up.

Katie said that she had found the procedures I had taught her quite useful. Swift was much more relaxed about her being close to him. She said that the face work had been helpful because now Swift was easier to brush and get a bridle on. It was also easier for Katie to deal with his feet because he did not keep picking them up. He was more supple when being ridden and she felt that the tail work had contributed to this.

Conclusion

I learned a lot about working with a highly nervous horse. It took about twenty minutes before Swift would allow me to begin the session. I had to be very patient with him and stay very relaxed. I performed rotations with his toe on the floor so as not to upset him and tried to avoid any situations that he may have found stressful.

Owner's comments

Linda Roe, Katie's mum, wrote the permission form. She said that Swift is a very sensitive and nervous pony and the shiatsu sessions have really helped to relax Swift, and given him a lot more flexibility in his muscles. He is a much happier and more trusting pony. 'Alison has been very helpful.' Linda said that I had explained the benefits of the work to her, she felt that her horse was in good hands, that 'Alison is extremely good at her job' and that she would recommend this as an ongoing source of help for her horse.

Student practitioner   Nicholas Goody

Horse Ernie – eight-year-old Thoroughbred dark bay gelding
Work Nil
Owner Heather Josh

History

Ernie had a bad fall in April '98 resulting in a twisted pelvis and being lame behind. He was rested all summer and came back into work in July '98, walked for six weeks and reshod to balance foot, then he became lame in front. X-rays and nerve blocks were inconclusive. The horse has been turned away for another six to twelve months with suspected deep-seated tissue damage. He is on one bute every other day and is not shod.

Personality

Happy, good natured, willing horse.

Session One – 9/02/99

Visual observation

When walked out, Ernie had short, choppy steps as though he had sore feet, looked balanced and mobile from behind and was obviously lame on both front legs as he turned. Lameness seemed to come from the shoulder.

Observation by touch

All-over stroking, Bladder Meridian. He was tender on the Bladder Meridian towards the quarters and became very fidgety when I worked this area on both sides. Gall Bladder: began just behind the right hand shoulder which was just a little tender at first. I moved back towards the quarters and he was very tender on the right hind leg towards the hoof and very, very tender in front of the shoulder moving up towards the head. Ernie became agitated when being worked on this point. He was a little sensitive around the ears but he accepted the work here.

I palmed the shoulders and found they were good except towards the front near the breastbone where they felt very solid and tender. Careful work did not relieve the sensitivity. I jiggled and palmed the neck; the problem is not in this area.

I quickly worked through the stretches and rotations which seemed to improve the area to the front. I returned to palm round the bottom of the shoulder and it was less sensitive but Ernie was still touchy. The front legs are very free and mobile in rotations and stretches so I concluded that I had not really stretched the area that was held in tension. He accepted the stretches and did not react during any of them. He seemed very flexible.

Hindquarters stretches and rotations: Ernie was very tense during these. He did not try to take his foot away but did not want to stretch at all. There was some marginal improvement as the leg was stretched forward but this was only marginal.

The tail was flexed and stretched; he did not stretch that much but there seemed to be no tightness or resistance. The back did not seem stiff during this technique on either side, just tense as though he was not prepared to relax. Body wipe.

At the end of the session, Ernie was looser and walked a lot better but still very tense. After the session, I felt there was a problem in the hind end and this was putting pressure on the front end.

Session Two – 25/02/99

Ernie was much looser and the owner felt he was sounder for two days following the last session but the stiffness returned. Still lame when walked in a circle on the walk-out, this looked the same as before the last session.

All-over stroking and Bladder Meridian followed by the Gall Bladder. Ernie fidgeted throughout and paid no real attention. I rotated and stretched the hind leg and he is, as last time, very stiff behind.

I decided to work on the Triple Heater because I felt it would be good for the shoulder pain identified last session. He reacted well to this at the top of the leg and around the eye. I then worked the lower part of Heart Constrictor by picking up the leg and working from the hoof to the knee joint. He reacted well to this by dropping his head and breathing more deeply. As I worked higher up the leg he relaxed more. I selected this meridian because it runs close to an area at the top of the leg that is very tender.

I then wanted to work on the area that was tender in the lower part of the shoulder at the front so I started wiping towards the area which he gradually came to accept. I palmed around the shoulders, being very gentle over the tender area. Followed with all stretches and rotations on the front and moved to work on the neck.

Ernie was tense, not stiff, towards the right so time was spent flexing the neck before returning to rotations and stretches on the hind leg to see if he could gain any more freedom. I then did hoof rotations. I then showed the owner how to work on the areas of pain around the shoulder and also to do the rotations on the hind leg to increase mobility. However, due to previous injuries, Heather is very stiff so the hind rotations were very difficult and she probably will be unable to complete them.

After the all-over stroking Ernie was walked out and was looser in the shoulders. Heather wanted to lunge him; the lameness was almost gone and she felt he had improved 60% on the right rein. On the left rein he was not sound but in the canter he changed legs and slipped. He was clearly trying to protect the right hind in the canter. She then stopped the canter and trotted him. The lunge session was not for work but so that she could see his paces.

I feel Ernie is lame in the right hind and it is the way he carries this leg that is upsetting his balance and promoting the intense shoulder pain.

Session Three – 2/3/99

Ernie was lame on both reins in the walk-out, perhaps not hobbling as much as last time but still noticeably lame. The owner has not been able to do any of the stretches since last time.

All-over stroking, Bladder and Gall Bladder. The horse was calm and did not fidget at all. After discussing the horse with Pamela Hannay, I stroked the front of the shoulders and watched where he was nipping. He was nipping at sensitive points that lie on the meridians where the Lung and the Large Intestine cross the breastbone. When I worked on either side of the Large Intestine away from the sensitive point in both directions, this desensitised the point. I kept my supporting hand on the sensitive area when working both the Large Intestine and the Lung Meridians, I then did all the stretches and rotations on all four legs. For this session Ernie actually offered his legs for the stretches, unlike previous sessions.

At the end of the session, Heather lunged Ernie again. On the left rein he was nearly sound and looking quite balanced compared to before at both walk and trot. On the right rein, Ernie walked as well as on the left but as soon as he was asked to trot he began to buck and leap. During this frantic session my attention was drawn to an area just behind the shoulder, so when he came back under control I worked from his pelvis forward to a point just before the shoulders and his right shoulder dipped away from my thumb at a point just behind the shoulder. This point is located on the Bladder Meridian. I then offered a tail stretch and, unlike the first session, Ernie really did lean into the stretch and the area on the shoulder moved. I did not want this checked by asking him to do any more work on the lunge and Ernie was therefore turned out into the field.

Conclusion

I have learnt that Ernie needs more regular sessions. It is not practical for me to work on him twice a week due to my own time commitments at this stage and the owner feels she is not capable of doing the shiatsu work as her body will not allow it. We have agreed that I will continue with weekly sessions for now. I can make a small improvement in three sessions but now understand that shiatsu is a long-term solution. The stretches can give short-term benefit but the complete treatment including meridian work is the way forward and this will not be a 'quick fix'.

Student practitioner   Jill Blake

Horse Scrumpy Jack – eleven-year-old part Thoroughbred brown gelding, 16 hh
Work Eventing, showjumping, hacking
Owner Sally James (signed and completed Permission and Evaluation form)

History

Jack is used for eventing and show jumping and enjoys going to these parties, but does not like schooling and puts in the most enormous bucks without any warning; he also does this when out hacking, so it is not a boredom problem. He is difficult in the stable, does not like strangers and is liable to kick sideways (which I was not told until after I had stretched his back legs although I had asked!)

He is hacked out regularly by his owner and ridden in the holidays by her daughter, Liza, who is away at university now. She is a rather nervous lady which I think communicates itself to Jack and I also think he misses Liza because he has become considerably worse since September when she went away.

Personality
Unpredictable and volatile.

Session One – 11/1/99
Visual Observation

On first entering the stable Jack was sulky and turned his back on me, so I decided to ignore him for a while and eventually he checked me out, found I was not frightened of him and stood with his head under my arm for maybe thirty seconds. I do not normally work on horses in a headcollar but I felt it prudent to be able to grab him if he did turn nasty. I used the usual opening procedure and found his left side very cold and unenergised. I later found out that he does not work properly on the left rein, and cannot do lateral work on this side. This would need stretching and balancing. He finds it difficult to stand square, and walks short on the off hind.

Observation by touch

I decided that I would use Bladder Meridian first to connect his back end to his front, then Heart and Lung. I also thought that touching on Liver 4 would help with the stiff hindquarters and his generally angry disposition.

Palming down the Bladder Meridian and then using fingertips was fine and he relaxed a lot, even yawning. I then used Heart Meridian which he was very curious about but felt I needed to take longer on the right (stiff) side. I worked the front and back of his shoulder, percussed the shoulder muscles and gave him a little stretch. He would not stretch and was unhappy, grinding his teeth and finally stepped forward deliberately onto me. This happened with both front legs. I then used Lung Meridian and after this he blew his nose and seemed a little happier to stretch. I felt he was trusting me a bit more. He seemed to like back lifts and they got higher with each one, also he lowered his head more and more and the space behind his withers filled out. I worked on his neck then, stretching and lowering and using Stomach Meridian on his gullet and jugular groove to encourage this. Now we had a very relaxed horse!

His hindquarters were very tense indeed on both sides, more particularly the right. He made no attempt to kick but instinct told me this was just below the surface. I worked Liver 4 and used percussion gently on his hindquarters with no ill effect, so I then stretched his hind leg backwards but he would not let me stretch it forwards. I did not attempt tail work for obvious reasons and felt that any more work on his back legs or hindquarters would upset him.

I then went to his head and he thoroughly enjoyed the face work. We finished off the session on this quiet note with the usual closing. He was very quiet, and I advised that he stayed in his stable for a couple of hours before going out into the field.

I suggested to the owner that she try some shoulder rotations, back lifts and stretching techniques on his neck – all the things that he had enjoyed – but not to upset him, and to do these, say, once every third day as part of a grooming routine.

Two days later she rang me to say that he had had a schooling session with a lady who is a BHSI and she reported remarkable progress. He was much softer and freer in his shoulder and worked very happily.

Session Two – 22/1/99

On reflection, I came back to Jack too soon. His owner wanted another miracle but he was not happy to oblige. He was very angry, although he greeted me well enough and we started as before with an opening session and Bladder Meridian. I just knew he was not in a co-operative mood and did not want to upset him further. I quickly worked on Lung and Liver after the Bladder but did not attempt any stretches to his legs. I worked on his neck, lowering and stretching and finished off with his face.

I then found out that the owner had been trying to stretch him every day and had had somewhat of a battle and eventually lost her temper. We had a long discussion about this because he is not a horse you can do this with, which she of course realised. I was quite happy to see him again but suggested a longer break before I came back.

Session Three – 3/3/99

A much happier Jack. The longer break between sessions suited him and I dealt with him exactly the same on the third as on the first visit. I used the same meridians as these had been of obvious

help first time around. It differed in that he was a much quieter horse and more co-operative, enjoying his front and rear leg stretches and allowing me to stretch his hind leg forwards and do plenty of tail work without threatening me. I made this a fairly quick session in order not to overdo things and make him angry. I felt he trusted me more this time. On his initial walk-out he swung along in a freer manner, especially the right hind, and on a midway walk-out he was very relaxed with a longer stride and Bladder Meridian moving nicely. I felt that he was much more in harmony with himself, and his owner said that he had been calmer and had not bucked since the first session.

Conclusion

This horse has taught me more than any other I have seen. He was so obviously angry, emotional and tense, which his owner could not recognise, maybe because she is a very emotional and tense person herself and this reflects in him. I have tried to teach her how to be more relaxed with him, to breath with him and find quiet moments in his life, and from the reports I have of a couple of happy hackers, this seems to have worked. She is very pleased and has recommended me to several friends whose horses I have seen. I did not know until ten minutes into the second session that she had been overdoing my suggested exercises: this came out in a confessional manner when it was obvious that he was resenting my attempts to help him. I will need to use this experience and relay it as a gentle warning to other clients. Enthusiasm must be controlled firmly.

Owner's Comments

Very much softer and freer in his schooling, particularly freer in his shoulder, happy in himself.

Student practioner   Liz Eddy

Horse Kizzy – twelve-year-old pony, grey mare, 14 hh
Work Pony Club
Owner Mrs Hilary Anderson (signed and completed Permission and Evaluation form)

History

Kizzy has a history of laminitis. She is ridden by Mrs Anderson's eleven-year-old daughter. Kizzy twisted a fetlock in spring '97 and was put on box rest for three weeks. At the end of this time she had developed laminitis. For the next nine months there were heart-bar shoes, foot resectioning and almost permanent lameness. Mrs Anderson called me because she felt Kizzy had become so depressed that she had lost the will to recover.

Session One – 20/12/97

Visual observation
Kizzy was totally miserable and absolutely crippled. It took her about ten minutes to walk twenty yards into her stable.

Observation by touch
Because of the laminitis, I decided to work Heart Constrictor and Triple Heater. To ease general pain and stiffness in the shoulders and back, I worked Bladder and because laminitis can cause hormonal upset in the horse, Spleen was worked.

I worked the back first to try to induce some feel-good factor; she relaxed a little so I started on the front legs. As the feet were very hot, I worked from the ground up moving from one leg to the other with thumb pressure and standing leg jiggles. On moving to the hindquarters, she kicked out when I touched Spleen 6, so I worked to desensitise the area for next time. On returning to the front legs, she picked one up so I quickly gave leg rotations and stretches. Her shoulders were incredibly tight but it was impossible to say if this was solely down to the laminitis or whether there was a tendency to tightness anyway (I would

guess it was the latter). I finished by jiggling the neck to try to help her relax.

As her feet had cooled a lot, we took her for a walk round a field and she moved with much more ease. I left Mrs Anderson instructions to jiggle the front legs, thumb-up the legs, jiggle the neck and palm the back, twice daily.

Session Two – 6/1/98

Kizzy is still crippled but much brighter and is walking more easily. This time I was able to rotate and stretch the hind legs (the backward stretch was gratefully received) and was able to do a little more with the front end to help the shoulders relax. I also worked the neck, especially Large Intestine. I worked the poll but felt I had to be careful as one of the side effects of laminitis can be high blood pressure so I did not want to make things worse. Kizzy was turned out in a small patch where she wandered off and rolled.

Session Three – 14/1/98

The vet had been back in between my visits so I got the evil eye from Kizzy who was now able to walk away from me! Everything just kept getting better and Mrs Anderson was now able to give rotations and stretches to all four legs. The neck stretches are improving. This time when turned loose, Kizzy started cantering up the field although she is still lame on hard ground.

Kizzy had two more sessions after this, by which time she was being ridden again for the first time in months. By the summer of 1998 she had returned to full work with no ill effects.

Conclusion

Patience is all and the language of touch can get through to horses better than anything else.

Owner's Comments

Kizzy had been ill with chronic laminitis for nine

months when Liz was approached for help. Initially Kizzy was reluctant to 'let go' as Liz worked on her but by week two had relaxed visibly. We were interested to see quite violent tail swishing and stamping of hind legs when the lightest of touch was applied to various points. This diminished (i.e. this reaction) as treatment progressed. By the end of her treatment Kizzy reacted like a different horse and was much more flexible in her movements. She enjoyed the sessions very much after initial resentment had worn off. We felt the sessions were extremely informative and that the horse was in good hands at all times. We would recommend shiatsu as an ongoing source of help but, hopefully, the condition will be managed so as not to recur.

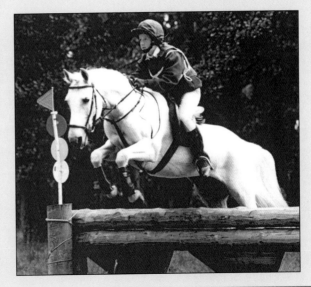

Practitioner and teacher   Jacqueline Cook – Level Three

Horse Bosworth Field (Bozz) – DOB: 1984, Cleveland Bay x Thoroughbred gelding, 17.3 hh
Work At present Bozz is in light to moderate work. Previously he had been hunting and done BHS Horse Trials to Intermediate standard. When he was unable to stay at this level he later did Pony Club activities with Liz's daughter.
Owner Liz Cousel
Case history date August 2000

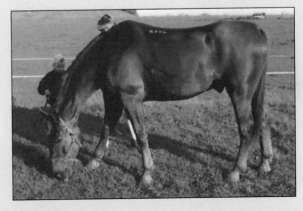

History

Liz Cousel has owned Bozz for fifteen and a half years. He lives in a rural DIY livery yard and is turned out with a 15 hh gelding. Other paddocks with a variety of horses and ponies in them surround their paddock.

Bozz had strangles at the age of five, he then developed Purpura haemmorhagica, with a 10% chance of survival. For the last eight years Bozz has had a lot of problems with his forelegs, with a variety of vets looking at him (many x-rays, scans, nerve-ending tests etc. done on him) and all giving a similar comment 'he's not lame, but he's not sound either'.

Body type
Bozz is a wood-element type, with more yang constitution than yin. His problems were very much in relation to his type:

General muscle soreness
Neck tension – headaches
Joint, tendon and ligament
    problems   yang – Gall Bladder
Circulatory problems
Hind leg stiffness
Muscle strain/inflammation
Eye problems   yin – liver

Session One

Visual observation

As Bozz was taken from his box to be walked out for me, my first impression was how bolt upright his head and neck were, with a tremendous amount of inflammation at his atlas/axis region which was transmitting tension and lack of elasticity further down his spine. His tail was clamped. He also seemed to be unaware of who or what he was standing on or over.

When moving at a walk he could not track up, demonstrating the lack of movement in his lumbar region and that his quarters were extremely weak. He was lame on all four limbs indicating the musculoskeletal and biomechanical function was under excessive stress. His circulation was also very poor.

Bozz's whole constitution was very depleted, visually you could see this particularly in his quarters where the muscle was showing deterioration, he was showing a reluctance to move forward and a lot of general fatigue.

Observation through touch

A session of shiatsu always begins with a hands-over-hands introduction, stroking the horse all over. This prepares the horse for a session and helps the practitioner to discover more about the horse, i.e. hot spots/places indicate inflammation (too much energy), cold spots/places (not enough energy, will often be seen as a weak area, muscle deterioration). It also gives the practitioner a chance to pick up any previously unseen lumps or bumps.

Bozz was very unhappy about being stroked all over, he was too sore to bear even this simple technique particularly around his poll region. His tail was rigidly clamped and his legs were stone cold. His hair was pretty coarse to touch where it was standing on end. His muscle structure would brace against the touch.

The main meridian pathways that I worked on with Bozz were:

Gall Bladder   For general muscle soreness, neck tension, joint, tendon and ligament problems, headaches.

Liver   For hind leg stiffness, circulation problems, muscle strain and inflammation, eye problems.

Bladder   For hind leg soreness and stiffness, neck pain, back pain, general fatigue, clamped tail.

The following points were used during Bozz's sessions:

Gallbladder – point 21   To relieve shoulder pain, soften tense muscles, used for hock problems.

Gallbladder – point 29   To relieve disorders of the hip joint.

Stomach – point 36   To relieve fatigue and help restore the immune system.

Stomach – point 2   Relaxes muscles, tendons and the body in general. Excellent pain relief point.

Large intestine – point 4   To relieve pain from any part of the body.

Bladder – (Large Intestine association point) point 25 Relieves pain in the neck, shoulder and lower back.

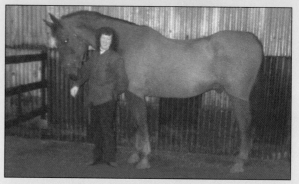

His first session was very difficult as his body was extremely sore and deep pressure could hurt him. I used only palm pressure at this stage, with soft subtle movements. He found it very pleasant and some relief was pleasing for him. He was unable to do any leg rotations and stretches at this stage.

It was after his first session that Bozz blossomed with the work. The tension and soreness eased, to be replaced with muscle that became fuller and the elasticity had returned within the whole body structure.

Bozz had to be shown how to move again as he had been compensating for so long that he was moving incorrectly according to his conformation. This was done through rotations and stretches, encouraging him to be aware of his body in motion.

Today Bozz is the picture he should be for his breed and size: a big, beautiful, powerful horse who has good active hock action, fluent movement and who is in control of his body, and is now sound.

Conclusion

In today's modern world the pressure to succeed is greater than ever; the equestrian world is no exception, putting a lot of pressure on horse and rider. It is very important that all practitioners work together to bring about the profound results and give relief from these pressures where possible. Bozz is one of many I see, demonstrating how beautifully we can all work together.

Owner's comments

In the last ___ years or so, there have been long periods when Bozz has not been quite sound. He has been x-rayed (by different vets) on several occasions. Apart from general wear and tear, nothing was diagnosed until recently when I was told he had mechanical laminitis. I was advised to avoid trotting him on roads and told he would probably have to be on bute indefinitely. I did not like this, so I asked Jacqueline to come and give me her opinion. Six months later, thanks to Jacqueline and her shiatsu, and my vet Sam who agreed it would be a good idea, Bozz is now as sound as a bell and looking better than ever before. Treatment will go on a while yet, but it has all been worth it.   Liz Cousel, Yate, Bristol.

Vet's report

Bosworth Field

Bozz was presented in June 2000 with a three-tenths degree of lameness at trot in his left fore-limb, with the toe area of the hoof being positive to hoof tester pressure. The area was explored but no infection was found, only mild signs of inflamed laminae. The lameness improved to almost sound with a bilateral abaxial seasmoid nerve block. The horse had a history of front foot pain a few years earlier, which had been improved with bar shoes, plus he had moderately poor fore-foot conformation with broken-back hoof/pastern axis, collapsing heels and flat feet. In the light of this, front foot radiography was advised to rule out any bony pathology.

Radiography showed no bony abnormalities, so bar shoes combined with low dose phenylbuta-zone were prescribed due to foot conformation and possible early mechanical laminitis. After four weeks (and off the phenylbutazone) Bozz's lameness had improved to sound on a straight line but persisted at three-tenths lame on the left fore on the left rein and one-tenth lame on the right rein. More time was given and further anti-inflammatory treatment given as well as keeping him shod with bar shoes.

Another month later and the left-rein lameness was persisting. The left foot was no longer sore to the hoof testers and it was beginning to look like Bozz was suffering from a secondary problem. His large size and unusual conformation of higher quarter assembly compared to front assembly with a weak back made it likely that past and recent lameness problems may have left Bozz with stresses and strains on various areas of his back and other parts of his anatomy.

Bozz's owner was keen to try complementary therapy and certainly something to help bring his body 'back in line' and working as a unit was indicated. Shiatsu therapy was suggested and we decided that we would see if it could help as conventional medicine had done what it could. Jacqueline Cook, a local Shiatsu with Horses practitioner, was contacted in August and Bozz has had regular sessions ever since. Bozz has steadily improved both in his lameness and physical ability as well as his mental attitude, becoming a much happier and relaxed horse, indicating a relief from pain. At his last check up in mid December he was sound on a straight line and on both reins on the lunge, as well as having built up muscle in areas where he was weak as a result of a gradual exercise programme suggested by Jacqueline to go along with her shiatsu therapy. Bozz still has his bar shoes on at this stage and these may eventually be removed only if the foot conformation improves sufficiently.

This case highlights well how conventional and complementary therapy can work hand in hand to improve and resolve a chronic lameness. This case resolved because of good professional communi-cation between all three parties involved, with each person having an open mind as to how to help Bozz and treating him as a whole horse with appreciation that a problem in one leg can have a knock-on effect on other body areas.

Samantha Stock B. Vet. Med, MRCVS (Rowe Veterinary Group, Glos.)

Conclusion

Thank you for your interest in this work. I hope you have found this book informative, enjoyable, challenging and useful in improving your relationship with your horse.

If you are interested in studying with me, please contact me for information on organizing a workshop or course in your area (telephone 973-927-0626). The following is a description of my three-level curriculum. The courses are geared to the needs of each group and each level is filled with practical information. You can experience a curriculum that focuses on self-development as well as practical knowledge of working on the entire body of the horse. I teach shiatsu for horse and rider (although you do not have to ride – I do not). It is a program that brings out the healer within each person. The techniques learned will enable you to develop a deeper level of communication with animals, and with people as well. The maximum number of people on these courses is twelve so that I can focus on each student.

LEVEL 1

Day 1 Students work on each other to develop proper use of their bodies, touching skills, feeling interpretations, and relaxation and centering techniques.

Day 2 Students work with horses and learn techniques for the entire body, including how to move energy in the meridians via limb rotation and stretching and meridian work. Practice is carefully supervised.

Day 3 Students finish studying techniques including the tail, neck, head and face. There is review time, and time to practice a full body session. Each student has a horse to practice on, however, some students prefer to work with a partner. I may suggest a specific procedure for each horse.

LEVEL 2

Day 1 We build on techniques studied in the first day of Level 1, with people working on each other. Students study some meridian locations, with techniques for feeling and interpreting what they are feeling, partner stretches and observation of body types, as well as kyo and jitsu.

Day 2 This is a review and refinement day, where techniques from Level 1 are studied in depth. Students are required to take turns demonstrating for each other.

Days 3 and 4 Each student will have time to discuss one case study they have done between courses. Meridian location, location of several points, and stretch positions of meridians are studied. Specific techniques for specific problems are discussed. Students learn how to decide which techniques to teach someone on whose horse they have worked. Each student will practice a full body session, with attention on what they hope to accomplish with a particular horse, and what they actually have accomplished.

LEVEL 3

Day 1 Development of a simple full body session geared to the problems of the rider's body, which must be balanced for the horse to be comfortable and happy. Exercises for the rider's body problems are taught.

Day 2 Morning hours are in the classroom where case studies will be discussed. Development of meridian theory correlations as they apply to the horse's body and mind in relation to the theory of kyo and jitsu will be studied.

In the afternoon I will demonstrate techniques and speak about what I am feeling, how I make a decision to continue to each ensuing technique, when to take a break and walk the horse, when to finish the session, etc. I will discuss the benefits of each technique, answer questions, and help students to understand how to use creativity and instinct. Students will have time to practice with these ideas in mind.

Day 3 Review day where all previously studied techniques will be demonstrated, as well as some new ones. Students will help each other with my supervision. We work on refinement of techniques and theory, with attention to stretching, movement effectiveness, students' own body mechanics, and connection to the horse.

Day 4 We will work on different horses from the previous day, who will have specific problems. These problems will be evaluated by us as a group and the horses will be treated. We will seek to hone our work to eliminate unnecessary techniques and get quickly to the core of the problem before the horse gets bored, uncomfortable or overdone. We will try to find the bottom line using our instincts, visual diagnosis, touching diagnosis, movement diagnosis and, lastly, the owner's evaluation of the horse's problem. Students will develop teaching skills to teach someone else techniques that may help his or her horse. Suggestions will be made for students who wish to do introductory demonstrations for others. Professionalism will be discussed.

Day 5 Exam day Students are required to demonstrate several techniques of my choice, and take a written examination.

Requirements for attending courses All participants must be fairly adept with horses on the ground and practice safe horse-handling techniques.

Prior to Levels 2 and 3, students must submit case studies of five horses, three sessions each, with owner's comments. Guidelines for these are supplied.

Certificates of completion are given at the end of each course.

Certification One year after the successful completion of Level 3, each student may present ten case studies on horses, and five on people who ride the horses. The student will demonstrate two horse treatments and one human treatment for me. This will be followed by an interview to discuss goals. Upon successful completion of these requirements, a practitioner's certificate will be given. This is renewable every two years following a demonstration of practical skills.

I also have arrangements and requirements for people who eventually wish to teach.

Details about courses at the Ohashi Institute in New York City can be obtained from www.ohashiatsu.org. Details about courses in the UK can be obtained from Jacqueline Cook BHS AI on 07721 739973 or 01367 718958, or from her website www.shiatsu-for-horses.com.

Index